MW01243057

Dedicated to:

SUSAN EIK FILSTEAD
because she is everything.

CONTENTS

ACKNOWLEGEMENTS

I had a few "false starts" when I would begin writing and reach a point where I did not want to go any further. Writing meant that I had to re-live, re-think, re-feel the experiences of sadness, anxiety and uncertainty that have come to characterize our lives. Yet for every aborted attempt to write the book, there was always a remarkable goal Susan was able to achieve or an obstacle she overcame—all providing a renewed sense of hope and resolve to begin writing again.

Susan's philosophy that "there may be a bad moment or a day, but it is not a bad life" brings a balance and normalcy to our lives. It is what sustains us when the efforts to push on seem futile. Her attitude and presence gives life to our lives.

Maureen Koertgen and Shelia Rigney have typed and retyped various drafts of this book. A thankless task given my penmanship. Their insistence on finishing what I started moved me along. I am grateful for their continued prodding. Ms. Gail Cates provided her editorial skills to shape my thoughts into complete sentences. If the story is clear, it is due in large part to her thoughtful comments and suggestions. Thanks to Jorie Epstein for preparing the final version of the manuscript. The fact that this book is available is in large part due to Tim Hotze. His efforts to bring the book into the light of day are greatly appreciated.

Ultimately, this is Susan's story—told through my eyes. I hope I have been able to capture who she is that makes her so special. It is her example of living that gives purpose to my life. Hopefully, others, unknown to us, can read this story and find the strength and courage to continue their fight, knowing that it is hope that sustains us all. Ms. Claudia West, Ms. Evelyn Sherrill-Ruffin, and Ms. Hannah Kushnick reread the manuscript for the last time. Their efforts are much appreciated and have added clarity to the story.

INTRODUCTION

Life is not easy. At times life appears unfair. Yet easy or difficult, fair or unfair, life goes on. We either engage it or life will surely pass us by.

On November 7, 2008 it will be 16 years since my wife, Susan, had an intracerebral hemorrhage the morning after our son, Matthew, was born. This is a story about determination and the human spirit, about a life-altering event and her efforts to reclaim her life. Her story is about thriving, not just surviving, about hope and not despair. It is a story of triumph and the reservoir of strength we all possess, to varying degrees, to overcome what seems impossible.

These are universal themes that most of us will confront at some time during the course of our lives. How we respond to the challenges we face will be the test of who we are. It is not the view from the mountain top but the journey to get there that makes the trip worthwhile. Striving rather than arriving is what makes one's life alive.

Susan's stroke and the subsequent development of intractable epilepsy have taken its toll on her physical and emotional health, but Susan is winning the war. She refuses to allow these conditions to define her or limit her opportunities. Susan has a disability but she is not disabled. To have the will to move forward in spite of the **DAILY** obstacles and challenges speaks to Susan's determination and resolve.

I was in a bakery last week and overheard a woman explain to the owner that she was having a small gathering at her home on the second anniversary of her son's death: "He would have been 21 this Saturday," she said. As she talked, she began to cry. She looked at me and said, "I'm sorry. I didn't intend to start crying. It's not easy losing my son." I replied, "That's OK. Don't worry about it."

We continued to talk when she stated: "People say I will be better in time. Time, they say, will heal my wounds." Without thinking through what I was about to say I blurted out: "Whoever said time heals all wounds never had a deep wound like yours to heal. It isn't going to get better." You have memories of what he accomplished, as well as expectations and hopes for what his future life would have been. It will never be easy to not see him graduate from college, get married, or have children. You have lost these experiences and the pain from these losses will always be with you. I hope you can relive and enjoy your fond memories of him, for your memories will sustain you and bring you comfort. Celebrate his life today since I'm sure he was a great source of joy for you."

I wondered who I was talking to. For sure her, but in some ways I was surely talking out loud to myself. The shock and sadness of that day 16 years ago; the losses Susan has experienced over these years and the uncertainties that lie before us are as painful today as they were back in 1992. Let me say that again. In spite of the passage of time, what has been lost and what will be lost in the future are very painful **DAILY** reminders of what we had and what we hoped for in our lives. These feelings are always present and I cannot imagine them ever going away or diminishing in intensity. But life goes on.

Susan lives with hope. Hope sustains her and our family every day of our lives.

Many individuals have encouraged me to write this book. Their belief that Susan's story contained lessons we could all learn from sustained me through these years. Our families have helped and supported us in ways too numerous to count. This journey would have been more difficult without them.

I began a diary as a way to save my mind. The idea of a book was never the impetus for starting a diary. Writing afforded a sense of pseudo-detachment from the reality of the daily events much like a reporter might "report" on the events surrounding a story. The only difference was this was not a story but our lives. Over time, in conversations with different people, it became clear that Susan's journey had value in telling. It was important to share with others the struggles and successes that marked the course she would take.

I considered writing about the events that have happened to Susan and me for some time. I find writing to be therapeutic—while I may not be very good at it, it does provide a vehicle to record events and reactions to them. You can say on paper what you may not wish to talk about—or ever say to someone else. Just because something is written, you don't have to share it with anyone. Nevertheless, this book began as a way for me to keep it together—now it's an effort to describe an event that would forever change our lives—and, ultimately, how we have come to make the best we can of our life together.

Stories typically have a beginning, middle, and end. This is the cycle of life. Yet, when one is living life, it is not always clear as to where one is at in this cycle. With hindsight, we have come to realize that the life we had ended the day after our son was born and the challenge is to find a way to begin again.

This story has no ending—we have just begun what will be a lifetime of coming to terms with what has happened. I seriously doubt if "coming to terms," whatever that means, can ever occur. What we knew and had has profoundly changed and what will be is unclear. This uncertainty is constant and exerts a sense of despair over the inability to control events or to plan for the future.

The only thing that is clear is that Susan and I are in this experience together and forever. So is our son, Matthew. We will find our way or, at the very least, enjoy the trip. It has taken time to get to this point of finishing this book—writing takes time and, as I would soon learn, time is a scarce commodity. There is also the pain of telling the story. Someone said, "If it's important, you'll find the time." I guess that is somewhat true. Nevertheless, it has become important to write, and the result is before you.

Pain—or perhaps profound sadness is a better way to describe feelings I often experience. To say this is not what I expected my life or our lives to be bears open the fallacy of this statement—if one knew in advance what one's life would be and what would be happening , how many of us would move forward but forward is the direction we clearly will continue to go.

--William Filstead
February 2010

A CALL TO REMEMBER

"We know what we are, but know not what we may be."

-*William Shakespeare*

Chapter 1: A CALL TO REMEMBER
November 7th - Saturday 8:00 am

"Mr. Filstead, this is Dr. Lee, the OB/Gyn resident at Prentice. Please call 312-908-5913 as soon as possible."

This is the phone message I received at 8:00 a.m. on Saturday, November 7, 1992, my 48th birthday. Little did I know at the time, how that call would totally change my life, Susan's life, and our lives forever.

I had just returned from a haircut and grocery shopping. My wife, Susan, had given birth to our son, Matthew, the day before. Susan suggested I get a haircut, so I'd look good for the first family pictures.

When I heard this message, my first thought was of Matthew. Something happened. I had talked with Susan earlier that morning, about 7:15 a.m.—so I knew it had to be Matthew.

When we had talked, Susan sounded very tired and sort of out of it. She didn't say anything about Matthew. In fact, I had called the high-risk nursery right before I talked with her. The nursery reported he was doing well—did well throughout the night—yet why the call?

Matthew was born early, at 35 weeks. He initially had trouble breathing. Lungs and lung development are always a concern with newborns. The pregnancy had been difficult for Susan. She was fond of saying, in her cynical way, "Do I have the glow yet?" She never had the glow! Susan was sick from the second month throughout the entire pregnancy. Her vomiting, euphemistically referred to as morning sickness, lasted throughout the day, everyday, and throughout the pregnancy. She had to be hospitalized early on in the pregnancy because of the vomiting and dehydration. Since Matthew was premature, upon his birth he was whisked away to the intensive care high-risk nursery. A team of physicians and nurses worked to get him breathing as soon as he was delivered. Matthew "had done well throughout" is what I was told a few hours earlier. So why the call? I was extremely worried.

As I heard the message, my stomach dropped. I didn't like the tone—sounded urgent—and the phrase "as soon as possible" made me very apprehensive.

It was 9:50 a.m., I had just missed the 8:00 a.m. call, and so I called back immediately.

"This is Mr. Filstead calling for Dr. Lee—I'm returning her call. Is she available?" She came to the phone.

"Hello, this is Dr. Lee."

"This is Bill Filstead calling. I got your message. What's the matter?"

10

"Your wife needs to go for a CAT scan and I would like
you to come downtown and hold her hand. Can you do that?"

"Sure, I can do that." I said.

"Good. Go to the 12th floor of Prentice. Ask for the head
nurse and she'll tell you where to go. Get down here as soon as you
can."

Don't ask me why, but I didn't ask why Susan needed a CAT scan. There was a feeling that it was needed or else she wouldn't be having it.

Rather than go downtown in the early afternoon with Alisa and Amy, my two older daughters from a previous marriage, which had been the plan, all of a sudden, there were ten things that had to be done and done quickly. I had to clean up, put the groceries away; but the first thing I did was call Alisa, my older daughter.

"Something happened to Susan and she needs a CAT scan,
so I'm going downtown right away. Let Amy know and I'll call you
later when I learn something."

I decided to call Amy directly. I didn't want one sister to feel the other sister knew more. I left a voice mail.

"Amy. Plans have changed. I'm going downtown now.
I'll call you later. Talk to Alisa about what you can do."

As I left these messages for Alisa and Amy, I recall being anxious and very worried. I tried not to let on because Alisa would wonder why the CAT scan. Worry, however, was the all-consuming emotion.

Faced with a clear choice – forward we move.

Chapter 2

GREAT EXPECTATIONS

"It is our attitude at the beginning of a difficult undertaking which, more than anything else, will determine its successful outcome."

- William James

Susan and I had worked together; my previous marriage was falling apart, and over time, I came to realize that I cared for her. On a summer day in 1981, since I was leaving my position at the University, I decided to take Susan out to lunch. Up to this point (we had known each other for two years), neither one of us had said anything or done anything that would have indicated feelings for each other. I had no idea what she thought about me, except that we worked well together—we got along.

I recall the days leading up to the lunch were an internal struggle for me. I wanted to say something, but I didn't know what to say. Should I say anything? Could I say anything? How big of a jerk would I be?

On that day, we walked over to this restaurant (The Palm) on Chicago's trendy lakefront. It was a warm summer day in July. The water was deep blue—there was a light breeze—and I was scared to death. I was still rehearsing words in my mind—over and over—but without any clear resolution. What was I going to do? It was difficult carrying on "small talk" while I had this internal conversation within myself dominating my every waking moment.

We enjoyed lunch, engaged in small talk, and as we were about to leave, I blurted out: "This may sound crazy, but the hardest part of leaving the University is leaving you."

The look on her face was one of total surprise—maybe stunned would be more accurate. I'm sure this was the last thing she had expected to hear, since she believed my marriage was fine. Furthermore, there was no reason for me to say anything. Surprised would be one way of characterizing her reaction.

After saying what I did, I truly can't recall anything else about our conversation. All I knew is that I felt good—Susan didn't laugh—and I did say what I truly was feeling. Whatever happened—time would tell.

Over the course of the next nine years, we lived together. I finally got divorced in 1989—one can easily see how "quickly I acted" and confused I was—but not about Susan. Despite my excuses, vacillation, inability to get it done, etc., Susan stuck with me. I am eternally grateful that she did.

14

We married on December 2, 1990, a lovely home wedding that Susan planned—I mean planned every last facet. Cakes—any type of cake is a weakness (or love, depending on your point of view, as well as weight) we share. Susan explored five to six bakers and tried cakes from each until she found a wedding cake that met her standards. My theory was, who cares (or eats) the wedding cake anyway? Susan wanted it to be memorable.

Having a child had been talked about on and off when we lived together and were younger. Time had passed quickly and at 37 years of age, Susan's biological clock was ticking (for all to hear). Since I already had two daughters, having another child was not my number one priority. As it became less and less an issue for me, it became a driving force for her. She wanted a child and, while I wasn't for the idea or enthusiastic - I wasn't against it. I recall joking that if we had no children, I could retire early and we'd travel and enjoy life (like the American Express ads) or if we had a child or probably children, I'd work until I dropped dead or was placed in a home, but at least the children could visit their father. We voted against early retirement and travel.

So, in the summer of '91, we decided to have a child. Having reached this decision proved easier than conceiving. As Susan had just turned 37 and I was 48, the biological/physiological processes, as the doctor said, "were shutting down." Since "getting pregnant" didn't happen right away; tests, examinations, procedures, etc. were recommended and tried. Susan finally became pregnant in April 1992.

This was the pregnancy from hell— uncontrolled vomiting, a hospitalization in the third month of pregnancy to control the vomiting and dehydration. About six months into the pregnancy, Susan began retaining water—she actually began swelling very early because she was unable to wear her wedding rings after the first month.

During the last three months of pregnancy, her blood pressure began to spike and she was spilling protein into her urine. As we soon learned, these were signs of preeclampsia. This is a high-risk pregnancy condition in which the body begins to reject the idea of being pregnant. The body doesn't like this idea, and both the mother-to-be and the baby pay a heavy price.

By October, 1992 (the seventh month), Susan had significant swelling in her hands, face, legs and ankles. Pictures taken at her niece's wedding showed how bloated and distorted her face had become. Susan was not on bed rest, but told to take it easy. "Sit down once in awhile and put your feet up. Don't shop all day—stay off your feet as much as possible," was her physician's advice.

Susan was already doing this. She did not feel good enough nor have the stamina to go all day. Being petite in size, she did not have a lot of room for the baby and her lungs.

In late October (the Friday before the presidential elections in 1992), Susan experienced the first and only pre-delivery episode of lightheadedness and spots before her eyes. She knew this didn't feel right and was concerned. But, the symptoms stopped and she went about her business.

On Monday (November 1, 1992), Susan called the doctor's office. They didn't get back to us until very late in the afternoon. The doctor's office suggested coming in for an evaluation, but we would never have made it downtown before the office closed (we live in a northwest suburb 25 miles out of the city). So a Tuesday afternoon appointment was scheduled.

Susan knew she was classified as a "high-risk pregnancy." Her set of symptoms were defined as preeclampsia. We were both concerned; Susan's mother had similar problems when Susan was born. But to be honest, we were not overly concerned.

Susan had been seeing her doctor for over ten years and had confidence in him. The hospital was rated one of the best in the country and certainly the tops in Chicago. She was doing all she could do to monitor her food intake and weight. In short, we felt she was getting the best care possible—there was nothing else that could be done that was not already being done.

Even though her due date was December 10, 1992, "her bag" had been packed for a month. The Tuesday appointment was at 2:00 p.m. I knew she thought I was crazy, but I suggested we take the bag along—just in case. It was only November 2, 1992, and our son (we knew the sex early on) still had five weeks to go.

We left the house, stopped at the park field house across from our home to cast our votes in the presidential election (Bush vs. Clinton) and headed downtown to the hospital/medical center. The doctor came into the examination room, engaged in small talk, and took Susan's blood pressure. He told her to lie down and he'd take it again in a few minutes. After the second reading, he said, "I want you to check into the hospital now—today—right after you leave the office, head over to Admitting."

She and I were surprised—very surprised! Even though I joked about taking "her bag" along, I never really thought we would need it. I recall our asking a host of questions in rapid-fire orderÖ

> *"How long will Susan be in the hospital?*
> *How was the baby? Is there anything to worry*
> *about—really worry about? Could we go home and*
> *check in tomorrow?*
> *What is going on? Why the rush?"*

The doctor explained that Susan's blood pressure was quite high, other signs like protein in the urine, blood work, etc., were not good and that preeclampsia is a serious problem. Then the doctor said something that neither of us has ever forgotten.

> *"My wife almost died of preeclampsia; if I*
> *wouldn't have intervened, she would have died. I*
> *helped her and I can help you."*

Things sounded serious (we didn't really have any idea what "serious" meant or how serious "serious" was). Clearly our plans had changed. Rather than go home, Susan was going to be admitted. I had a feeling that the baby would arrive shortly – not in five weeks.

As she was getting dressed to leave the doctor's office and head down the street to be admitted, her doctor stopped by to say that he'd see us over there late afternoon or early evening. He had called in orders. The nurses and residents would be getting things started.

As we walked over to the hospital, we both had the same sense of "can you believe this is happening?"—after all these years together, talking about having a child—the time had arrived. There was a feeling of anticipation and excitement with concern in the background. We were excited!

Upon admission, Susan was sent to a high-risk floor. This unit helps patients who needed extra monitoring or care. Once settled in the room, residents, nurses, medical students, lab technicians, etc., went in and out asking questions; each group repeating the same set of questions. Susan was hooked up to a blood pressure monitoring device; urine output and other vital signs began to be monitored hourly. Given the high level of activity and the bed rest order, we suddenly realized that there was concern for Susan's health. As the nurse said, "You have a very high blood pressure reading. If you stand up suddenly, you could faint and fall—we don't want any accidents to happen."

When we worried, most of the worry was about the baby and how early he would be (about four to five weeks before the original due date). Susan had read a considerable amount and was aware of the problems related to premature births. Would he be okay? Would there be problems because of the early delivery? Were his lungs developed enough? If he was too young to be delivered, would Susan be hospitalized for the rest of her pregnancy?

That evening, her doctor came by. He explained that all tests indicated the baby was okay and would be okay, but that he might have to spend a few days in the high-risk nursery. "He will do fine!" was the doctor's assessment.

Susan, on the other hand, had to deliver. Her health was a problem and would deteriorate if she didn't deliver. The treatment of choice for preeclampsia is delivery. There could be some seizures, but there was a crash box in the room that contained all the necessary drugs and/or equipment to treat such an eventuality.

"Just hang in there over the next few days, and you'll do fine," was the other reassuring remark by her physician.

18

Monitoring, testing, monitoring, and more testing was the order of the day and on into Wednesday evening. The plan was to monitor Susan and the baby to make sure both were okay.

When I arrived on Thursday morning (November 5, 1992), the plan was to deliver the baby. Various medications were started. All I could do was watch and wait—monitor, watch, and wait. That evening, the doctor told us the baby was going to be delivered on Friday (November 6) one way or the other. Either naturally, which he thought would be the case—or if problems developed—by cesarean section.

Susan's blood pressure was high, but within range given her condition. Nevertheless, these high blood pressure readings were the key symptom that necessitated the early delivery.

Magnesium sulfate was started to reduce the possibility of seizures. When I left Thursday night, I gave her a kiss and said, "Tomorrow you'll be a mother." "And, you'll be a daddy again," she replied.

With the advantage of hindsight, I'd have to say we were not overly worried. There was no reason why everything would not be okay. We had been reassured by her physician that "all would be right." Susan was in a hospital—being monitored. And not just any hospital - the premier women's hospital in the Midwest. This is sort of like the preflight announcements on airlines: there is the oxygen mask, the floatable seat cushion in the unlikely event of a water landing, exit doors, etc. Most hear it—few pay attention—all feel there will be no need for any of these devices.

This is how Susan and I felt. Sure things could go wrong, but it was very unlikely. Besides why worry about bad possibilities that haven't happened?

On Friday (November 6), I got up and went to the YMCA like I normally did. Played racquetball and let the morning rush hour wind down. Susan had an uncomfortable night and her water bag was broken about at 2:00 a.m.

I arrived at about 9:30 a.m. and discovered she had been moved to a labor/delivery room. Susan looked tired but was pumped. This was the day!

Lori, our nurse, made sure we knew where everything was; told us to get comfortable, and explained that because of preeclampsia, she would be monitoring Susan's blood pressure closely. The digital automatic BP readout unit was not working, so the manual pump-up BP/cup would be used.

A fetal monitor unit was strapped across Susan's stomach to keep track of the baby. After about 30 minutes, Lori told us she was going to talk to her supervisor. Susan needed to be closely monitored, and Lori could only take care of Susan, no other patients.

Blood pressure was the worry. Susan's was elevated (as expected) and was spiking (going up/down occasionally)—not a steady pressure. The stress on the baby was increasing as well. Labor was moving along, although when you are experiencing it, nothing seems to be moving along. You'd like it over with and it is unclear when that will happen.

By 2:00 p.m., twelve hours after the water bag had broken, delivery was getting close. Contractions were more intense, closer together, and Susan was dilating. Susan's physician, nurses, other doctors and residents were all coming and going throughout the morning. This pace seemed to quicken after lunch. At this point in the early afternoon it was a steady stream.

Susan's doctor called the neonatal intensive care unit to bring up a high-risk monitoring cart. They arrived (two doctors and two nurses) with a cart that had a heat lamp over it. Various tubes and monitoring devices were hooked up to the cart. They plugged it in and said they were prepared for the baby when it was born.

At 2:49 p.m. on Friday, November 6, 1992, Matthew was born—he didn't cry and was immediately taken to the cart. The neonatal team barked out orders and commands and worked feverishly. I was numb and very worried. No one said congratulations or you have a healthy baby boy — nothing! Despite the noise associated with all the activity, it seemed very quiet. I watched them work on Matthew and held Susan's hand. Still no cry. You'd like to know what is happening, but nobody volunteers any information—or if they know, nobody is saying

anything. We were too afraid to ask for fear we will learn
something we did not want to know.

Finally a cry! Not exactly a yell or an ongoing series of
cries, but a cry nevertheless. Matthew was immediately taken out
of the labor/delivery room and was on his way to the high-risk
nursery. The doctors who worked on him assured both Susan and
me that he <u>would</u> be all right (not that he <u>was</u> all right). I could go
down and see him in about an hour after "we have him hooked up
and stabilized." Not exactly encouraging words.

Neither Susan nor I felt good about what had just
happened. We were extremely worried. The worry and
apprehension grew by the moment. Susan, for her part, was
drained and had a "killer" headache. She did very well during the
delivery, but her blood pressure remained high following
Matthew's birth and her urine output had dropped. These
symptoms persisted.

Lori, the nurse who had been with us all day, suggested we
relax (what a ridiculous idea that was) because there was no hurry
to get back to the room. "I'll stay with you and we'll make sure
you're okay before we take you back upstairs. You'll get better care
and more monitoring here than you will up on the floor." Lori told
Susan.

Susan didn't feel well—so why rush if it was not necessary.
Susan and I, despite the pronouncement that Matthew would be
okay—while never saying so, had the same thoughts.

> *"Did something go wrong during delivery?*
> *Are his lungs developed enough?*
> *Was there—could there have been—any brain damage?*
> *Why didn't he cry—and when he did cry, cry so weakly?"*

Neither Susan nor I had really seen him or held him. She
delivered our son and he was taken away. It's easy to say to
someone, relax—when it is not you that has to relax. Or to "be
positive," when there is nothing to be positive about. We were
independently thinking the worst, because there was nothing that
happened which would have led us to think otherwise.

21

After waiting 30 minutes, I told Susan I was heading down to the high-risk nursery. I wanted to see him, hold him. I wanted to talk to someone who would ease my mind, our minds. I wanted good news. I needed some information to allow me to believe he was okay. Somebody <u>please</u> remove my fears! Our fears!

When I arrived downstairs at the nursery, I had to complete various forms about who I was and who would or could visit Matthew. There are a host of rules that have to be complied with. I was told to "gown-up" (and put on rubber gloves) before I was allowed to see Matthew. A nurse met me and led me over to his isolate.

Matthew was 4 lbs., 7 ounces, at birth and he looked like a little chicken. All skin and bones, with this breathing tube taped in his mouth. Lots of tubes, IV lines, monitors—he was sleeping, at least that is what I told myself. I preferred to think of him sleeping rather than in a coma or some other altered state.

The doctor who was in charge of the unit, along with one of the doctors who took care of Matthew in the labor/delivery room, came over to talk to me.

"He is doing very well. There were initial problems with breathing, but he is doing most of his own breathing now. We have cut back on the machine and my guess is that he'll be taken off of it in an hour or two."

"So he's going to be okay?" I asked.

"Oh yes. Being early and the medications always have an impact. But he is fine. He will have to learn how to swallow and gain some weight. We also want to make sure his lungs are okay and nothing else happens. He'll be here for about two weeks, but he'll be fine—don't worry."

"Thanks. Thank you very much for taking care of him." I appreciatively replied.

I did feel relief, but I can also say that I didn't feel 100% confident that all would be well. I still had a notion that there was a problem and I just didn't get the full picture—yet.

Knowing Susan would want to know about Matthew, I went back up to the labor/delivery floor. It was about 5:30 p.m. and her doctor was standing in the hallway.

"How is Matthew doing?" he asked.

"They said he was okay, but I'm worried." I said.

"Well, he'll be fine, I talked to them. I'm more worried about Susan—but we will watch her and she'll be going up to the room shortly."

To this day, I don't know what he meant by the phrase, "I'm more worried about SusanÖ" He walked away as he said that, also saying that he would check in with us later.

As I walked into the labor/delivery (L/D) room where Susan was, she asked, "Is he okay, what's going on?" "He's fine," I said. "He's doing real well." I didn't want to really say what I thought—saying "he was fine" would at least help her feel better about Matthew and his health.

Susan's blood pressure was still elevated. Lori had decided to stay beyond her shift just to be on the safe side and make sure everything was okay. Susan's urine output was still down and Susan's headache was intense. The lights in the room were dimmed; a cold rag was placed on Susan's forehead and Lori said, "Close your eyes for awhile. We will go upstairs when you feel better."

Residents and other nurses came in and out—looked at various outputs from the monitoring machines and said very little. Collectively, the message from all of these nurses and physicians was, "We just want to make sure you're OK." To me, these remarks meant Susan was presently "not ok." So I wondered why she wasn't ok and what could be done to make her better.

Around 7:00 p.m., a resident stuck his head in through the door and asked Lori some questions. Lori gave him Susan's blood pressure readings and urine output and asked, "Is it okay to transfer her back to the floor?" "Yea, go ahead. She's okay," responded the resident.

To us, heading back to the floor was good news. It had been a long day and Susan wasn't feeling well. Lori suggested we should stop by the nursery so that Susan could see and hold Matthew. Susan was excited by the prospect of being able to see and touch Matthew. She had yet to see or hold him.

Lori configured the bed and the monitoring equipment, IV lines, etc., and we pushed the bed down the hall to the private set of elevators that went directly to the nursery.

The nursery had been alerted to accommodate our forthcoming visit. As Susan's bed was pushed over to Matthew's isolate, the nurse moved Matthew closer for Susan to see. To my surprise, he no longer had the breathing tube or the machines, or all the IV lines – just one IV.

The one IV line inserted in his nose and taped to his cheek turned out to be how he was going to be fed. It was a gavage tube. Milk in a syringe is attached to the end of the tube and the milk went directly into his stomach. Until the sucking reflex developed, this was how Matthew would be fed.

Susan attempted to sit up, but was too dizzy. She tried to rest her weight on one elbow as she leaned over the railing of her bed to try and touch Matthew. But that didn't work because Susan complained of being lightheaded and dizzy. Her headache had not lessened—all she was interested in or able to do was lie down and bury her head into the pillow.

Lori, sensing that this was too much for Susan to take, suggested we head up to the room, get something to eat, get some sleep, and told Susan, "You'll feel a lot better tomorrow." We headed toward the elevators which took us back to her initial room on the 12th floor, the high-risk pregnancy floor.

Just like in a relay race, Lori "passed off" Susan to the nurse who would help us on the 12th floor. It was about 7:45 p.m. and the nurse on the floor took various system measurements and offered to get a tray of food so Susan could have something to eat. The hospital had some elaborate birth celebration dinner package, but that was out of the question. Susan wanted something light to eat—and to get some rest. Crackers, Jell-O and juice, three institutional staples were ordered and quickly arrived. I helped Susan change into a pajama set she had brought from home. She wasn't interested in eating very much, although she did try the juice and Jell-O.

Around 9:30 p.m., still feeling sick, tired, and with a pounding headache, Susan suggested I head home to get some sleep so that I could get up early, get a haircut, and head back downtown for pictures on Saturday. Funny how things happen. Matthew had been born on November 6, 1992, the day after my sister's birthday and one day before my birthday.

"Get some sleep. Take some Advil; maybe you'll feel better with some food and sleep." Susan seemed to agree with what I had said, so I headed home. When I got home, I called to see how she was doing and to let her know I had arrived home safely.

> *"My head still is killing me—I took the Advil awhile ago, and I'm going to bed. See you tomorrow. Love you."*

> *"I love you, Susan. You'll be fine. Matthew will be fine, and will be home in a few days. We can go downtown to feed him until he comes home. But we are doing okay. Quite a day. I'll see you in the morning. Love you."*

26

Chapter 3

THE NEWS

"At the core of life is a hard purposefulness, a
determination to live."

- Howard Thurman

November 7, 1992 - Saturday

Less than 30 minutes from getting Dr. Lee's call, I was leaving the house heading downtown to the medical center to see what was wrong with Susan. My adrenaline was pumping—I was wired and trying to do two or three things at once.

It was construction season in Chicago (we have two seasons, winter and construction) and the most direct route, the Kennedy Expressway, was under construction. As I left the house, I put the radio on to hear about the traffic. Just as I was about to head in on the Kennedy, the traffic report indicated it was backed up, so I took the alternate route (the toll way to the Eisenhower Expressway, then into the city).

As I drove, I replayed in my head what Dr. Lee had said, "Your wife needs a CAT scan. Can you come down and hold her hand?" I knew things weren't right—but I couldn't even comprehend what was wrong or how bad things could be.

I drove faster than the legal limit, was in a hurry. I knew I didn't need a ticket, but I also knew by the sound of Dr. Lee's voice that I needed to get downtown quickly. I recall thinking, "Christ, we were out of the woods, weren't we?" After all, Matthew was doing better and the real concern regarding Susan's health was the period prior to birth and the health of the child. What the hell went wrong?

I arrived at the hospital and parked right in front; went directly to the front desk and told the attendant:

> *"My wife had a stroke. I was told to get down here quickly, so I'm going to leave the car here for a bit."*

> *"Okay," she said, "but this is a baby hospital—she wouldn't be here. She'd be somewhere else.*

> *"I know, but I'm going to start on the 12th floor where I was told to go and see what happens."*

No one had used the word stroke in any conversations with me. I vaguely knew this was a possibility, but really had no idea what a stroke was. Think of how many medical terms we use: open-heart surgery, hip replacement, shoulder surgery, etc. You know, but you don't really know. The word just does not have any context—any grounding—any experiencial base so that it actually means something.

I was mentally trying to make sense of an overwhelming uncertainty. As I headed towards the elevators, people passed by, but they were a blur to me. I saw signs and activities of others, but they appeared blurred as well. Nothing is very clear externally to you. Internally, your mind can't shut off. It keeps asking questions that I struggled to fathom, let alone answer. I was downtown at the hospital, but why? Something happened, but what? What could happen? I was in high gear and felt it!

After leaving the sign-in desk, I headed down the hallway behind the reception desk. The elevator took its time arriving. After waiting for what seemed like an eternity, a bank of doors opened and I boarded pressing #12. When the doors opened on 12, I headed out onto the floor towards the nurses' station. As I approached, a nurse came towards me.

"Mr. Filstead?"

"Yes."

"I'm Colleen."

"What's wrong—where is Dr. Lee? She called about my wife."

"Your wife had a stroke. She has been taken to NICU (Neuro Intensive Care Unit) at Olsen. I'm very, very sorry."

"What a nightmare! You've got to be kidding. Jesus Christ, what the hell happened?"

(Then I started thinking why did she say I'm very, very, sorry!)

"Your wife had an intra-cerebral hemorrhage (bleeding in her brain). They transported her to the ICU and I'm to take you over there."

"Okay, let's go!" I said.

It is hard to describe the rush of feelings and fears that enveloped me. Stunned – numb – disbelieving – afraid – fearful - worried. There are truly no words to describe the emotional shock caused by the word stroke. I had never been in this type of "feeling state" before— or since—nor do I ever want to be again. Physically you are present, but mentally absent.

Olsen Pavilion houses a variety of services for the hospital. The two principal services are surgical suites and intensive care units. All the various pavilions are connected with above ground walkways. Having been on the faculty at the medical school, I knew my way around this facility.

When we arrived on the NICU floor, we walked down a long hallway at the end of which were two windowless doors with a huge sign above the doors that read: "Staff Only / Patient visiting hours on the hour at 9, 12, 3, 6, 9, and 12, for 15 minutes only." As the nurse and I approached, these doors automatically opened and a man walked towards us.

"Rick will help you now. Best of luck. Hope she's okay." With those words Colleen left.

Rick, a nurse on the unit, simply introduced himself and told me to follow him. He was going to take me back to cubicle #1724.

The floor Susan was on consisted of three separate ICU units. We had to walk down a long hallway, make a few turns, and walk straight ahead to the ICU area (as the sign at the entrance proclaimed).

Each cubicle had a person in it that looked either half alive or half dead, depending on your optimism or pessimism. The area was rectangular in shape with the cubicles arranged in a u-shape around the nurses' station.

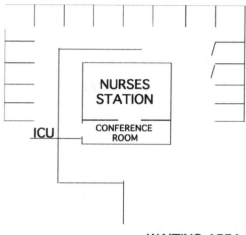

WAITING AREA

The area was very busy, even though this was a Saturday morning about 11:00 a.m. Nurses, technicians, doctors—every shape, size, color, were all moving in and out of the area. Patients were being moved down the hallway. Family members were visiting. There was a lot of activity.

As we walked down the hallway and passed the various openings, my eyes kept searching for #1724.

As I approached the nursing station, I saw a crowd of individuals standing in and immediately outside the unit #1724. Rick asked me to wait while he went toward the group.

A few minutes passed and the group, almost en masse, backed up and a short, Latin-looking individual emerged from inside the room and led them towards me.

*"I am Dr. Jost Biller, a neurologist, and I
have been asked to evaluate your wife and help care
for her."*

*"Hello. I'm Bill Filstead—nice to meet you.
Thanks for your help."*

*"Come with me. I want to explain to you
what happened to her and what we are doing."*

"How is she doing? Can I see her?" I asked.

"Sure, but come with me first."

He and I, followed by a group of six to seven other
doctors, nurses, medical students, etc., headed down the hallway
towards a conference room located behind the nurse's station.

Dr. Biller put her CAT scan films up on the view box. He
pointed out things as he talked. It was very weird to be looking
inside Susan's head.

*"Your wife has suffered a massive—a
massive bleed/stroke in her right parietal lobe area.
She is completely paralyzed on her left side, blind in
her left eye, and has no sensation on her left side nor
has any idea that she has a left side.*

*Her kidneys are failing and it goes without
saying that she is quite sick. Pressure is building up
in her head and I am very worried about her brain
stem."*

That is about all I could understand; I comprehended
some of what he said. What I didn't understand, I was not sure I
wanted to. It was a nightmare, and that was the phrase I kept

saying over and over again. It's a nightmare; a nightmare; a nightmare.

"We just had a baby—she has never seen or held him." My comment was directed at anyone who wanted to respond. I wondered if she could or would ever—given what I had just heard.

There was no feeling, no pain—a numbness, an emptiness—it was all-consuming. There were intermittent floods of thoughts—like scrambled data transmissions. "What did she know? Is she alert? What should I say? Would she recognize me? Could she talk? Would she die?" All I had were questions with no answers.

Dr. Biller said, "Too many questions with too few answers." Susan, according to Biller, knew she had a stroke and knew she was paralyzed—but did not really comprehend what it all meant. Who could, I thought! No one goes from being OK to being paralyzed and "gets it" right away. Think about it. Even if you try to move and you can't, do you think you are paralyzed? How do you grasp that you can't move? I had heard enough. Enough talk, I needed to see her.

As I headed down the hallway to see her, Dr. Biller stopped me and looked me in the eyes saying, "Be strong for her and you—things will be alright. Approach her from her right side, she will not see you on the left."

He walked with me up to the opening of her cubicle and stopped as I walked towards her bed – from the right side as he suggested. Susan was laying in bed with numerous lines, leads, catheters, IV's, oxygen, etc., everywhere. I have never seen so much machinery, readouts, electrical wiring, etc., in one small place hooked up to one person.

"Happy birthday, Bill! Can you believe this?"

I started to cry and so did she. "Well now that we've shed a few tears, what are we going to do about this fuckin' mess? We need to get out of here!" I said.

*"Right. This is a fuckin' mess. What are
they going to do?" she asked.*

*"I don't know, dear. The doctors are
meeting and trying to figure things out. I'm going to
go find them so I know what's up—I'll come back
and we can talk about it."*

"I'm scared Bill—real scared."

*"So am I. But we will get through this. We
have a lot to live for, and we will overcome whatever
has happened. Just remember—we are in this
together—you and I, till the end of time."*

"Thanks, honey."

As I left to find Dr. Biller and the other doctors, I told her,
"Don't go away, I'll be right back." Our black humor was already
starting. It was the only way to handle the pain and it would
become, over the years, a primary way for us to get through
whatever we had to. Joke about how bad things are—and it
becomes a joke. If you can laugh—even make fun of yourself—
you can survive. Once you stop or can't laugh anymore, trouble is
surely ahead. Anything that can mask the seriousness of the
situation – for a short time – defuses the situation.

Susan had all her marbles—she knew it was my birthday.
She surely knew the mess she was in. Fear, uncertainty, the
unbelievability of the situation—a rush of confusing and
overpowering emotions pressed on my chest. I knew now what
heartache felt like.

"Don't be long, Bill." Susan requested.

*"I won't—make sure nobody hurts you." I
replied. (As if anything else could happen.)*

Susan had tubes and monitors everywhere: an IV line, a catheter, oxygen mask, heart monitor, etc. I have no idea what it must be like to be hooked up this way—to realize it—and to realize the seriousness of the situation. She needed every line to live.

I had taken my phone book with me when I left home. I knew that I would be making calls and I was prepared. Susan's mother and father were planning to visit her and Matthew. I wanted them to know what happened so they wouldn't drive downtown. I wasn't sure they could handle it.

Before I left home, I had called my sister, Betty, to tell her I had to go to the hospital quickly. I asked her to call my daughters, Alisa and Amy, and bring them down with her.

As I left the cubicle Susan was in, my mother and her neighbor were standing outside waiting for me. "What happened, Bill?" she said, and started to cry. I just couldn't get any words out—just shook my head and cried as well. We talked a few minutes. This would be the first of many explanations of what went wrong.

Everyone I tried calling was not home. Finally I reached Susan's niece, Carole. Carole was overwhelmed by the news: disbelieving, destroyedÖ Carole said she would call whomever she could and also get in touch with Susan's parents.

The distance from Susan's cubicle to the waiting area was about a half a block. These points were at the opposite ends of this large, seven-story building in the medical center. Having worked at the medical center for years, I knew my way around the facility. I never, ever thought I'd be using or needing these facilities. I would soon learn that the walk up and back provided quiet and peaceful moments for reflection, for thinking, for planning whatever we had to do to get better.

I told my mother and her friend to wait in the family area while I went back to check on Susan. Each walk allowed a lifetime of thoughts and experiences to pass by. There were also the immediate life-threatening concerns, as well as the future—but the future seemed impossible to contemplate. All that existed and mattered was NOW—what to do now. Now even seemed like a long time.

This "back and forth" between Susan and the waiting area would become a standard routine. Only two people could visit her at a time and the nursing staff wanted me to control the flow of people. Since it was a Saturday, it was not as busy or crowded in the waiting area as it could have been. Only emergency surgeries are done on the weekend.

I really don't recall who began to arrive first —Susan's brother and his wife (Chris and Joyce), my daughters (Alisa and Amy) and sister (Betty), her parents (Otto and Viola), her niece (Carole) and her husband (Jim), friends, etc.

Everyone wanted to know what happened? Everyone wanted to see Susan, but this was not a time for visiting. Susan was in an enormous amount of pain from the bleeding in her head and her medical condition was critical. Having a parade of people come and go—or worse, stay and try and talk, seemed impossible and not helpful.

I recall someone saying "but I want to say goodbye." I told them not to worry since Susan wasn't going anywhere. Yet that request jolted me – she could die. I had considered this reality before but not in any serious way. Now hearing "I want to say goodbye" made this possibility more plausible.

In talking with her father and mother, I used a profanity in discussing Susan's situation. That set her father off on a religious tirade. He is a born again Christian, but believes that only he and the handful of members of the church he attends are the chosen ones. Only they really know. Both he and Viola were very upset, so I didn't think it was the time or place to erupt, but that time would come soon. I just tried to calm them down, explain what had happened, what she looked like, how sick she was, and to approach her from the right side, since she had no sight out of her left eye. Her parents could not grasp the seriousness of the situation which was just as well.

There is nothing one can say to someone in Susan's situation that has any substance; small talk is meaningless. Platitudes such as "it will be all right" are ridiculous. People who say such things don't know what to say. So whatever is said makes them sound foolish. If you don't know what to say – best to say nothing.

A crowd was gathering, and I decided it was best for Susan not to have people coming and going all the time. I'd come back to the visiting area and give updates when there was new information. Family and friends would stay there and wait. That's what Susan needed.

While family and friends were gathering, the doctors were deciding what to do. Dr. Biller, the neurologist, had already paged a neurosurgeon to have him convene his surgical team. Northwestern University was playing Michigan in college football that day in Evanston, north of the city. The neurosurgeon, Dr. Brem, was attending the game until he was paged to come to the hospital. He arrived about 3:00 p.m. in the afternoon. I found out later that members of his surgical team had also been called prior to his arrival. It was decided that there was no other decision but to operate. All were scheduled to arrive shortly.

Dr. Biller asked me to step out into the hall to discuss things with Dr. Brem.

Chapter 4

SURVIVING – JUST SURVIVING

"My strength lies solely in my tenacity."

- Louis Pasteur

"Your wife is extremely ill. She has suffered a massive intracerebral hemorrhage that occupies a quarter of her brain and is pushing on the remaining parts of her brain—and her brain stem. We'd like her to be more medically stable than she is, but there is no time to waste. Dr. Brem and I agree that she needs surgery immediately in order to save her life. She will die without it. Do you understand the gravity of the situation?"

("Yes I do, I certainly do. So what are you proposing to do?")

"We need to stop the bleeding and evacuate the hematoma (blood clot)," said Dr. Brem. In a factual and straightforward, yet profound way, he went on. "As Dr. Biller has said, this is a massive bleed. That she is alive, has survived, and has her faculties is a miracle. She is paralyzed on her left side. With any luck, she'll regain her sight in the left eye, will probably be able to walk, but I'm not sure how well—but will have profound problems with her left hand and arm. There will probably be cognitive deficits, but the scope and severity of these problems are difficult to gauge."

"I will cut a hole in her skull, more like a 3x3 square, and remove the blood, and repair what damage I can. This is a straightforward procedure that I have done many times. I don't anticipate any problems. The only difficulty is to do this as quickly as possible. Pressure is building on the brain stem. We need to do the surgery now before there will be no need for the surgery."

The calmness in his voice and his factual approach gave me a sense of confidence. Hearing what I did left no choice—surgery with all the risks or death if we delayed – yet I felt an overwhelming responsibility for her life. I wanted to make sure, as best as I could, that this was the right and only thing that could be done.

I wanted to know what he (Dr. Biller) would do if it were his wife. "Surgery. There is no other option. She will die if she doesn't have this operation. This is her only chance." Therefore, we had to take it.

This decision was reached at about 3:15 p.m. the afternoon of November 7, 1992. It would take a while to assemble his surgical team, but Dr. Brem felt that 5:00 or 5:30 p.m., the latest, would be the time of the surgery.

I went back to the waiting area to assemble the group so they all could hear—I only wanted to say this once—what the plan was. I think the idea of surgery was not unexpected, but the phrase "brain surgery" was hard to fathom. Any type of surgery seems undesirable, let alone brain surgery. Since there was no other option but surgery, I was very glad that at least there was an option – and one with hope.

Everyone wanted to go back and see her—sort of like a paying of the last respects march. Nurses didn't want that, I didn't want that, and speaking for Susan, how would you feel if everyone came in to say their good-byes—no way.

I stayed inside her cubicle explaining to Susan what was going on, while family and friends looked in and passed by from the outside. There was a lot of activity going on to get her ready for surgery and to be able to transport her to the OR with all the lines and IV's she had stuck in her.

Jasmine and Rick, her two nurses, were thoughtful and kind. They were always with her doing something to her: pricking, pulling, taping, sticking, etc. A swan catheter was surgically placed in her neck and threaded down into her heart. This would allow for close cardiac monitoring.

Susan and I talked—hard to believe she was alert and able to carry on a conversation with all that was happening and how bad she was feeling. She had an excruciating headache from blood building up in her brain; she had dry heaves; wanted water, but couldn't have any. Talking passed the time, it occupied our fears so we did not have to think about them. As the pain increased I had her squeeze my hand.

Both she and I were very positive about the anticipated outcome. We had confidence in the doctors and she—we—needed a break. Something had to go right, and it might as well start now.

We talked about our lives, what we did, planned to do, fond memories, hopes—all the while people walked in and out all around us. Our private lives and thoughts were now public, but we didn't care. We were oblivious to what was happening around us as we talked.

"We should have done a Living Will like I wanted to," said Susan.

"We don't need one. Besides, we don't want to talk about such things at this time. Not a good omen. We don't have anything, anyway, so there is no need for a will."

"You need to promise me that you'll 'pull the plug' if things turn out badly. And, you'll take care of Matthew. I don't want to live if I can't have some type of livable life. Promise me!"

"Sure. Don't worry about it. I promise. Does that make you feel better?"

"Yes. Thanks."

"You know promises can be broken."

"I know. But I know you'll do what's right for me. I know you will. I trust you."

"You're right."

"I love you, Bill. You are the best thing that has ever happened to me."

*"Keep this up and we'll all be crying. I love
you, Dear. Remember, 'til the end of time—you and
me."*

Clearly, in my wildest dreams I never, ever, dreamt I'd be
having such a conversation with Susan. Other people have these
problems—you hear about them all the time. And you wonder,
what in the hell are they going to do—can't imagine what I'd do.
Well there is no time to imagine, we are the ones having these
discussions.

Between 3:00 and 5:00 p.m., the pace of activities picked
up. More nurses and doctors. Family and friends still arriving and
briefly visiting. Susan was getting worse—so the fewer the people,
the better. Her kidneys had practically stopped functioning. The
headache was beyond "on a scale of 1 to 10."

I had talked things over with the extended family. We
were all positive—hopeful—but what else could we be or should
we be? Who in their right mind would look on the bleak side of
this and project the worst-case scenario. It is natural and reassuring
to believe all will be all right—whatever that means. There is really
nothing else to believe. Hope and optimism sustains you.

Funny as it may sound, Susan and I tried to joke about
things as she awaited surgery. Discussed the fact that the surgeons
voted for Bush (Clinton had won the election), but we still trusted
them. Joked that we would have preferred a Democratic surgeon,
to which the surgical resident assisting on the case responded, "I
think you want someone who knows what they are doing, no
matter how they voted." Could tell this guy had no sense of
humor.

Talked positively about the results we expected. I made it
a point to stress over and over the fact that things would be all
right. We would get our lives back. I recall saying:

*"Don't believe anything negative someone
tells you. You will get back your life—our lives.
Walking will be possible. They are wrong about your*

arm—but forget it. It doesn't matter. You're young and determined. That's what counts. We need to believe and not listen to any of their pessimistic projections. Time and effort will tell, and you will work like a dog to get back who you are, what we had, and what we want for the future."

Throughout this ordeal—at least up to this point—I had had my moments, especially making the long walks back and forth between the waiting room and Susan's cubicle. But I surprised myself by how focused and composed I had been. I was bound and determined to be strong and positive for her—for me—for us. We needed to believe and be united in this belief.

By 5:00 p.m. it was time for surgery. The pace quickened. Susan's bed, with all the lines and monitors had been made portable for the trip to the OR. She had nine lines, plus oxygen. We kept talking in spite of the activity, other people, and the noise. Nothing else was important, so we kept talking. Never thought I'd ever be in a position to hear and say "last good-byes." I was bound and determined that would not happen.

Susan again said, "I want you to know again that you are the best thing that ever happened to me."

"So now you tell me—finally! Why are we talking like this anyway? Things will work out—you have to believe that. There is just too much going on and things to live for to stop now."

Again, she made me promise, and I promised not to let her linger brain dead. But, I quickly added, "Now with that small formality over, can we get on with our life?"

It was now 5:30 p.m. and it was time to start rolling to the operating room. There was real concern about the brain pressure build-up and damage to the brain stem. If that happened, it would be all over.

I walked along side her bed, holding her hand, as the bed rolled down the hallway towards the elevators which would take us to the OR floor. We knew this was a life-threatening situation and we chose to focus on life, rather than the threat.

Nurses and doctors came along for the ride. "Wait on the 7th floor," the resident said. "We'll take her from here. We have to get going." I bent over and gave Susan a kiss, "Don't cause any trouble. I love you. Remember, 'til the end of time." ("Love you, Bill.") And they pushed off behind a set of large gray doors. Once those doors closed there was absolute silence. I could hear and feel myself breathing – like I needed to catch my breath. A sense of being alone and helpless overwhelmed me.

As the doors closed, I had a feeling of confidence that everything would be all right as all right could be, given this circumstance. I also knew that whatever would be, we would deal with it. It was not going to destroy us.

Yet, at the same time, I felt lonely and apprehensive. A five-hour surgery is a long time to wait—but wait we will. How did this happen? Plans! The future! There was no way to comprehend these big (or little, for that matter) questions. Here we were—what was next? Whatever was next was the only thing I could concentrate on. We just had to wait and see.

I took the elevator back to the floor where the waiting room was located. Wanted to tell everyone what I knew and what the timetable for events was. As I got off the elevator, I met Susan's best friend, Melinda, trying to board the elevator. Melinda was out running errands throughout the day and I had not been able to reach her. On her own, she had planned to come down and see Susan and Matthew. Upon arriving at the maternity hospital, she was directed to the Neuro Intensive Care Unit. Having been a radiology resident at this hospital, Melinda knew that something had gone terribly wrong—just what, she was not sure, but it had to be catastrophic given the location. Ironically, Melinda had been at the same University Michigan (she's a graduate) and Northwestern football game that the neurosurgeon, Dr. Brem, had been attending.

"Where's Susan? What's wrong? Why is she over here?" All good questions and when I gave her the answers, Melinda was devastated—she cried uncontrollably. In her wildest dreams, just like mine, she would never have expected this. It is unheard of. Who would think that a blessed event could almost be deadly.

Each person to whom I explained what had happened to Susan made the telling of the events much more difficult. It was like reliving the bad news over and over again. To have to keep repeating the story added to the bizarreness—it truly was a nightmare.

Given Melinda's past residency experience and contacts at the hospital, she was able to go behind the scenes, check in and find out what was happening: at what stage was the surgery? Was progress being made? Was Susan tolerating this surgery? This stream of information turned out to be a great help and a source of comfort, since no information is almost unbearable. It's hard enough to wait and know nothing—as the wait lengthens, the waiting becomes more and more difficult.

Having about twenty people gathered in the waiting area, someone decided it was time to eat. Some wanted to go out and eat, others suggested bringing food back. Others were engaged in small talk (Carole and Jim had returned from an exotic honeymoon to Bali). I chose to walk up and down the hall. Pacing was a helpful activity. I didn't want to leave the building in the event something happened or the doctor finished early. Knowing what had already happened, who knew what else could occur. I just didn't want to leave. Besides, I had no appetite.

No matter what we talked about or how much pacing I did, time dragged—it did not move. As the hours passed the sense of anxiety increased. Memories flashed before me. I was present physically and then again, mentally, I was in my own world.

Every once in awhile, her dad, Otto, would approach me with "God will cure all evils, if you just believe." He wanted to know "if I believed." "Don't bother me" was my response.

I had caught him saying prayers over Susan while she lay in pain in the ICU unit before her surgery. I told him that was the one and only time he was ever going to do that. If I caught him doing that again, I'd never let him see her again.

Melinda had gone over to view the CAT scan. I pressed her for information. She said, "It (the bleed) was very large/significant," She volunteered, "I have never seen anyone survive such a bleed; since she did, that was a good/hopeful sign." Knowing Melinda, it was probably worse than she was saying, which gave me a sense that this was as bad as it could be. So we waited. Waited! No other choice but to wait.

Originally the surgery was planned as a four or five hour operation—in by 6:30 p.m. and out by 10:30 p.m., but we all knew that a lot can happen to affect this timeline. Dr. Brem said he'd send out periodic updates to let us know where things stood.

Time passed and at about 9:00 p.m., some of the group was going out for a walk/drink/cigarette. I felt it was too close to the surgery ending to leave, plus there had been no real updates. I had expected someone to say, "Things are going well." Also, Matthew had to be fed. I was making trips over to the nursery to feed him every two to three hours. If I didn't go, somebody in the group went or eventually the nurses fed him, if no one showed up. At 9:30 p.m., a nurse came out from the surgical area to get me, because she said Dr. Brem wanted to talk to me. I remember meeting him in a hallway outside the OR.

> *"Everything went fine. She tolerated the surgery well, has lost quite a bit of blood and received and will receive more transfusions. We shaved her head and opened up her skull with a 5x5 inch hole. I would guess we extracted the equivalent of three large eggs (tissue) and fluids that could fill a Coke can. Aside from the bleed, there was no obvious structural or vascular damage."*

> *"With luck and time, recovery will occur. Just how much of what, in what sequence is unclear. I don't believe she'll ever have the use of her left arm and hand. She'll probably be able to walk with some assistive devices. However, when I say walking I*

47

*don't mean like you and I walk. She will be able to
ambulate." (I have since learned that ambulate is the
medical term for walking which in no way resembles
what everyone else means by the word walk.)
"Cognitively she should be ok, but I really can't say
she will be who she was with all her faculties."*

A relief! A load off my shoulders! Such trite phrases don't
capture the "thank God she's alive feeling" I had when he (Dr.
Brem) began talking to me. I can't really put into words what I felt
or how I felt. People aren't prepared to experience these events, so
a true sense of uncertainty/unsureness marks such a conversation.
Also the emotions are magnified since such an event does not occur
often, if ever. Thus, the feelings are truly undefinable. To me, the
only words I want to hear were "she survived the surgery." All the
rest we can deal with.

In some ways, all of these events, the unexpected early
hospitalization, the difficult delivery, Matthew looking frail and in
trouble, the bleed, the reality of the stroke, the surgery, etc., had
numbed me to feelings—any feelings. I knew I was relieved and
joyful to know Susan was alive and that the prognosis was good,
but that just didn't seem like it was enough. Sounds greedy, but I
wanted more. I wanted Susan to be like she was. I wanted
someone to tell me it would be all right—would be like the old
days. I wanted to wake up and realize I had been dreaming—none
of these things happened. No such luck. God only knows what
Susan's first thoughts would be if these were the thoughts I had.

The phrase "she is young and time will tell" translates to
"she won't ever be the same, but what you'll get, you'll get. We
just don't know what that will be."

After hearing this news, I went to the waiting area to let
everyone else know. Tears of joy and relief—lots of tears. Our
families and friends had come to support Susan and me, as well as
each other. It was great we could all get a little good news before
many of them headed home.

There was no sense in everyone staying overnight. It was
now approaching 11:00 pm and many of those who had been

48

waiting had been here for 10-12 hours. Susan's mother was going to stay until she could see her and then stay downtown with Carole and her husband. Melinda and I were going to stay overnight; just to be around if anything was needed.

The group, minus the above, headed home. There was nothing more they or anyone else could do. I was told it could be midnight or 1:00 a.m. before Susan would be coming down from surgery to NICU. At 4:00 a.m., Susan was scheduled for a follow-up CAT scan post surgery to evaluate the operation. Would the brain reoccupy the cavity? Would there be any bleeding? If so, would the blood reabsorb? Would she have any use of her left side? Lots of "woulds."

November 8, 1992 - Sunday

The wait for Susan to return to the NICU seemed longer than the surgery itself. I received the first words at about 9:30 p.m.; it was now 12:30 a.m., Sunday morning (six and a half hours since I let her go through those gray doors). I was pacing in the hallway, when I saw this bed, a group of individuals, and all sorts of equipment and apparatus come rolling down the hall towards the NICU. It had to be Susan. I really didn't think there would be anyone else undergoing brain surgery late Saturday night.

As the bed approached, I could see that her head was wrapped with a drain tube taped to the side; she had a full-face oxygen mask that was forcing her to breathe; there were lots of tubes, medication lines, and monitoring lines with readouts on a set of screens that were hooked to the headboard. I was surprised someone could be moved with all this equipment.

Betty (her night nurse) asked us to wait a few minutes until they were able to get her settled and hooked up in the monitoring cubicle. We complied (Melinda and I), but stayed by the door so we could look in and see what was happening.

I had more questions than answers occupying my thoughts. Would she be awake or unconscious? Could she talk? What about her marbles? Would there be any cognitive impairment? What about the left side? What could she do or feel? What about a ventilator? How hard was it for her to breathe?

49

When Betty signaled it was okay to come in, the apprehension and anxiety heightened. I approached on her right side, since she could not see out of her left eye prior to the surgery.

"Susan, how are you doing?" I hoped she had heard me, understood what I had asked, and would recognize me. After all the time we had spent together, would she even know me? More fundamentally, was she Susan, the person I knew and loved? She opened her eyes and smiled. "I have a lot of pain, but I'm okay, I think." What a joy and relief—she was Susan. She was alert, had her marbles, could talk, etc. She looked a mess and the physical setting contradicted her statement of being okay, but it was good enough for me. If she thought she was OK that was all that mattered.

Susan had no sense of where her left side was, or that she even had a left side. Her vision from the left eye was impaired. Lying in bed was all she could do. So what! At least we knew what we had and could go from there. After all it had only been a couple of hours since the surgery.

Melinda and Susan's mother briefly said hello. They wanted to see for themselves that she was all right. There was no need or intent to visit. I just wanted Susan to know we were there and would be staying overnight. If she needed anything, a nurse knew where to find us.

It was close to 1:00 a.m. The follow-up CAT scan was scheduled for 4:00 a.m. Rather than nap (too pumped to do so anyway) I decided to go feed Matthew. I wanted to hold him and tell him Mommy was okay. He had to get to know Mommy, but it would be some time before they were both up to it, especially Susan.

This medical center is a large complex covering a few city blocks. However, most buildings are connected by above street ramps (two of them between the main buildings) or through underground tunnels. It was about a block walk to where Matthew was. At 1:30 a.m. or so on a Sunday morning, there are very few people around—it is as if I was alone in the complex.

Everyone at the high-risk nursery knew about Susan and what had happened. They had made accommodations to allow the

50

group that had gathered to see Matthew—also to have multiple family members feed him—given the extraordinary nature of the situation.

Matthew was tiny—4 lbs., 7 ounces, and dropping—all babies lose some of their birth weight. My daughters had been 8 lbs., plus—so he was certainly on the small side (okay for his age), but small to handle.

He looked fine, not as scary as when the tube was taped to his mouth. When I first saw him, I expected someone to drop the other shoe and tell me that he was in serious trouble. But that was not the case. The doctors and nurses on the crash cart had accomplished their task of getting him going, making him stable, and allowing him to rest comfortably.

My mind was racing with thoughts and doubts as I cared for him and did what I was suppose to do. As I fed him I told him Mommy was all right—started to cry—the emotions were just overwhelming. The uncertainties, doubts, fears, hopes all ran together, and now there was the real and added responsibilities of caring for Matthew and Susan. Being alive was Susan's first step—getting as healthy as possible was the next; being a Mom would happen in due time.

I walked back to the NICU waiting area. I had arranged the chairs and sofas into "bed-like" configurations. Melinda had already fallen asleep. I tried to, but mainly I tossed and turned.

Over time I must have dropped off, when suddenly I heard this voice calling my name. At first, I didn't realize where I was, but I quickly remembered what had happened and why I was sleeping in the family surgical waiting area.

It was Betty, Susan's night nurse. She wanted me to talk to Susan. "Your wife is refusing a unit of blood and she wants to talk with you," said Betty. Betty had told Susan it was time for another unit of red blood. Susan, concerned about AIDS, refused. What Susan didn't know is that she had lost quite a bit of blood during surgery and had already received four units.

"What's the matter, honey? Betty tells me you won't let her give you a unit of blood."

"I don't need to get AIDS on top of everything else. That's scary!"

I told her, "Dear, you already received four units while in surgery. Susan, you need the blood. Let Betty give it to you." Susan had an "oh shit, you have to be kidding me" look on her face.

Then she said, "Okay, fine. Give me the goddamn blood. But if I get AIDS, I'll put a gun to my head and blow a fuckin' hole in the left side to match the hole they made tonight. I don't believe it."

I started to laugh. Susan never swore like this, it was out of character, though her blunt and colorful characterization of her predicament was accurate. Betty overheard me laughing and asked what was so funny. I told her, and she said, "Being able to think like this six hours after brain surgery is a good sign of recovery."

I went back and told Melinda who also had a good laugh.

I fell asleep for about one hour when Betty reappeared to tell me that it was time for the 4 o'clock CAT scan. I woke Melinda and we both went with Susan, pushing her bed with Betty and talking as we walked.

This was a good time to visit, since there was a walk and there is always a wait no matter what time of day. Also, Melinda could play doctor and see the CAT scan as it was being done— most importantly she could interpret it on the spot.

"Good news! The scan looked fine; no bleeds and the remaining blood was reabsorbing. Everything, at least as seen from the CAT scan point of view, was where it should be at," said Melinda.

This trip up and back to the CAT scan area and the scan itself took time. It was 5:30 a.m. when we arrived back at NICU. Matthew was scheduled for another feeding at 6:00 amÖ.so off to the nursery.

He is so small and it is so lonely in the newborn ICU. Even though the nurses do a great job, it's not the same as Mom and Dad fussing over him and holding him not just at feedings. You pass people in the hallways or see individuals in waiting rooms and you wonder what their story is. They, like me, wouldn't be here if there were a choice. What tragedies are they confronting? Who knows?

I also realized that our partnership would probably undergo changes—was not real clear as to what it all meant—would have to wait and see until Susan got back on her feet. In spite of the conversations I was having with myself, it was real clear to me that our lives had been changed profoundly and forever in ways we only would know about in time.

There was also the realization of Matthew. Susan couldn't be a part of his life at this important time in both their lives—no holding, feeding, caring for him. Even though she was in enormous pain and in and out of consciousness, she always asked about him—and she herself realized and felt the loss of not being with and seeing him. Knowing Matthew needed her, and realizing she had more need than Matthew and could not help him now was very difficult for her. It added a burden that was only truly knowable and felt by her. I simply reminded Susan that she was the Mom and would do what Moms do when she could.

It was approaching 7:00 a.m. I was planning to go home and clean up when my family arrived. My sister called to say she'd bring down a change of clothes and shaving stuff, so I didn't have to go back and forth. That turned out to be a good idea.

By 9:00 a.m., Sunday (almost 24 hours after the bleed), people began arriving; both sides of the families, friends, etc. (must have been 25 people). Everyone was real pleased with the outcome and happy that things had turned out so well. When death is a distinct possibility surviving is one indicator that "everything went well" – whatever that means.

You sort of have to stop and think a minute, as Susan was fond of saying, "I didn't die, but I felt like I was dead." Don't get me wrong, there was joy in her surviving this catastrophic event, but at the same time, it devastated her, her life, and her hopes and plans. As each moment passes, the joy of surviving wanes and the concerns about the here and now grow. Surviving is old news. What do today and tomorrow hold? Where is the good news about the future?

Like the old saying, "you wake up one morning and it's a whole new ball game"—well Susan woke up and realized the game as she knew it was over or at the very least had significantly changed. What could she do to get her life back? What kind of life would it be? No one really knew the consequences of what had happened, but everyone was happy. We were all so elated that Susan was alive!

Then there was Matthew. Everyone wanted to see Susan and see Matthew. So I designated Alisa, my older daughter, to be in charge of the tour groups; the grandmas, sisters, etc., could go over on tours and take turns feeding him. The nursery usually wanted only one individual designated to take care of the baby. Such a rule cut down on unwanted traffic. However, our situation was unique and they were very accommodating.

Trying to see Susan presented problems. This was an intensive care unit with strict visiting hours, so a parade of well-wishers was out of the question. Steve, her nurse, made it a point to put an end to the cycle of visitors because it was out of hand. Susan could not handle it.

She could not tolerate the visits—the medications, the pain, trying to talk with an oxygen mask and tubes—impossible. Chris, her brother, had a great idea. Get a Polaroid camera and take pictures of everyone and Matthew. This was so she could see him and how he looked. It was the best we could do; he couldn't visit and Susan wasn't going anywhere soon. Pictures were a great idea.

Melinda also had a great idea. She purchased a charm from Tiffany's in which a picture could be placed. Took a picture of Matthew and placed it in the charm, pinned the necklace to Susan's gown so that she knew where it was at all times. Without a doubt, holding onto the locket got Susan through many days and nights.

November 20 - Friday: 7:10 a.m.

No real time to write all weak, too many things to do. No time for anything. Sounds all too familiar—no time. Time will be in short supply from here on out.

Some highlights:

Susan was able to move her upper left arm and close her left hand—not a real hard fist, but a good sign that functioning is here and we can build on it.

Matthew is coming home on Saturday, great for him—tough for Susan. This has been weighing on her mind for the last few days. She realizes this is going to be a difficult separation. We will have to figure out ways to make family visits, to be a family.

This is why we did this—got pregnant to have a child. Not being able to go home as a family is extremely difficult, but we will get over it. It's difficult to see Susan grieving over her inability to take care of Matthew as she had planned. I can only imagine her feelings of not being able to take him home; of staying behind after we leave.

My mother came down yesterday to practice taking care of Matthew. She did a real good job, even gave him a bath. I think she surprised herself about how capable she was.

Matthew is doing real well. Amy and Alisa will help bring him home. Funny how all of a sudden they are the big sisters. Glad they love him so much. Clearly, this is a change in their position from when they first heard about the pregnancy. They were not exactly excited about the possibility of another sibling. "You are too old," they reminded me. Old or not, here we are.

Every event has multiple meanings. Susan was able to move her left leg. A simple task before the stroke and a heroic act after the bleed. However, compared to the initial paralysis, the movement of her left leg was unbelievable. So, do you always use your past as the comparative standard—or do you use what you did last? There is no answer for this; we do both. With luck, down the line, both standards will become one. She will be what she was and then some. Remembering what we had–what she had–will stop.

Susan had a big decision to make about a requested angiogram of her brain. Dr. Biller and his crew were in last

55

evening trying to give us their perspective on things and what they'd like to do. More tests. They'd like a brain angiogram to make sure there was no underlying structural or vascular damage that happened to get worse and blow with the stress of pregnancy. We talked about whether or not Susan should do this—whether this is "overkill" (excuse the pun)—what could be gained from it versus the drawbacks?

Not an easy decision, since it involves the head. However, we balanced not taking the test with the future doubt about every headache to come. We don't want to live with a major doubt over what had gone on in Susan's head. To always wonder if a headache is a harbinger of another stroke is too much to bear. If there is a problem it has to be fixed.

Obviously, a stroke is a possible adverse consequence of this procedure. While explaining these risks, Dr. Fernandez, a fellow working with Dr. Biller said, "Öit's a very slight risk." My thought was how slight was the risk that Susan would have a stroke after delivery? I wonder how many women have had brain surgery following preeclampsia? What are the odds? So clearly, we were worried that our luck was not exactly going in the right direction and wondering whether lightening could strike twice. Needless to say, we hope not!

I talked to her mom and dad. I also called Melinda. She is going to come down and be with us, as well as check things over. It's a comfort to know she can double check the films, the orders and the treatment strategy.

I'm glad I came down to the hospital early—Susan is worried—don't blame her. But, at least, she and I can worry together.

Too many calls to make, people to keep informed. Everyone wants to know the latest as it is happening. It is impossible to make all these calls so I don't even try.

My secretary is going to start a Monday newsletter which will summarize what has gone on, what is planned, and where things stand. This info sheet can have a wide circulation which will reduce the number of daily calls.

November 21: Saturday, 10:20 p.m.

Matthew came home today—that's the great news! Susan stayed behind. That's the devastating news! In a nutshell, that's the day. A very bittersweet experience. It is hard to believe one can be so happy and so sad at the same time. This conflict of emotions makes it difficult to feel anything – to actually enjoy Matthew's homecoming. It is a profound sadness – one that probes your essence. It is a feeling I felt when Susan had the stroke – never before. But it is an all encompassing feeling of emptiness, of loss; it is a void that is painful – palpable almost unbearable.

I got up about 6:00 a.m. to try and straighten the house and get things ready for the big "homecoming." Took Hans, our German Shepherd, to the bakery, to get bread and a "Welcome Home Matthew" cake. When I went to pay the bill, Laura, the owner of the bakery, said the cake was on her. Can you believe that! I was truly touched by her generosity. I ran around like a chicken with its head cut off (not a good analogy)—lots of things to do with so little time.

The girls (my daughters, Matthew's sisters) arrived at our house around 10:15 a.m. to help in bringing Matthew home. They have been real sweet and concerned. I wouldn't have expected anything less. They are good kids; they understand the differences between their mother and Susan. They can love them both without feeling guilty about it—a mature lesson to comprehend at their age, or perhaps at any age.

Amy is real sad about this. "I'd trade places with Susan so she could come home." No better example of her love. Alisa is also very concerned and doesn't want me to worry about her tuition or anything. Like I said—good kids!

Getting the car seat organized and in the car was a project. It has been a while since I tried to attach a car seat. I learned that car seats have changed in the past 18 years. I needed a graduate degree from MIT to figure out how to install it. Maybe that wouldn't even be enough. Once we got the "carrier" separate from the base unit, we put the unit in the car, another gigantic undertaking. Nothing is simple with all these contraptions. I felt a sense of great accomplishment in finally securing the car seat until I realized I would have to go through this entire process downtown as we prepare Matthew for the ride home.

I encountered construction traffic and arrived one hour late (noon, instead of 11:00 a.m.). When I arrived, Susan said she had fallen this morning and hit her face while reaching for something on her bed stand. Why was she left unattended? Why did she reach? Could she judge her spatial surroundings? Anyway, it happened—but no real damage—at least I don't think there was.

Susan needs assistance in getting "dressed" – changing from a hospital gown to a t-shirt and pajama bottoms. I tried to help her get a bra and a T-shirt on. This was demeaning for Susan—to be helpless and struggling while trying to retain some semblance of privacy and dignity is the cruelest fate. We struggled, but got dressed. Bra and T-shirt over the hospital gown, no pants or anything. The original plan proved to be too complicated. "Just cover me up" became her fashion tag line. So I wrapped a blanket around her and helped her into the wheelchair, ready for the long ride to see Matthew. Susan could barely comprehend what was happening. Her head is pounding. Her heart is broken. It is less than two weeks since major brain surgery. Standing is impossible. Other than these and other "minor concerns" (the list is extensive) everything is fine. Carole, Susan's niece, arrived, so we all headed to the nursery for his big send off – minus Mom.

One good thing about being late is that there was no one left in the nursery to go home but us. A few of the nurses who cared for Matthew came by. There was a note on his crib to Mommy.

To say the note was a tear-jerker is putting it mildly. Paraphrasing, it said:

> *"I love you and will miss you, but Dad will take care of me until you can come home. I'll miss you, but will be thinking of youÖYou're the bestest Mommy, Love Matthew XXOOXXOOXX"*

Someone took the time to be thoughtful enough to help us through this tough time by writing this note. It was heartfelt but it not only broke but shattered what remained of Susan's heart.

We fed him. Susan held him and I propped up the bottle. We changed him into his going home finest—and prepared to take him home. Susan was physically present but seemed distant. The drugs, recovery from surgery, and the pain of seeing others get him ready to go home as she was staying behind were too many assaults on her self. Too much to acknowledge. Mom went with us to the lobby where we loaded Matthew into the car. The girls stayed with Matthew while I went back inside to be with Susan.

I took Susan back to her room. One of the longest walks I can remember. You could see and feel her pain. It was palpable. Our pain. Going home had arrived. Now, she is deprived of this unique experience. To make it more painful, she has never held Matthew with both hands, bathed him, fed him by herself, changed him, comforted him, and may never, unless her arm gets back to what it was. She can't ambulate, meaning she cannot walk. There is no possible way Susan can hold him and walk. Standing and transferring from the wheelchair to a chair takes extraordinary effort.

I sometimes wonder, does she even comprehend what is going on? How clear is her thinking? This is not real clear to me. All of these experiences are taking place in uncharted waters. Does she even know what to know? How much more pain can she endure?

Susan and I talked about the joy and sadness of the day, a very difficult conversation. So here I am leaving Susan, at one of the lowest points in her life, because Matthew is in the car ready to head home. I have to take him home. Susan should be coming with us. Just another example of what lies ahead.

Amy and Alisa watched over him until I returned to the car. Carole stayed with Susan. We headed home to a family welcoming party: Joyce, Pat, Betty, Bobbi, Vi and Otto, etc. (the family) was waiting. I had set up the house before leaving to get Matthew and they brought the lunch meats, etc., for a luncheon. There was a banner on the garage door, "Welcome Home

Matthew"—pictures galore—and Matthew loved every moment. He was wide awake, content, and very alert. Obviously a party boy from day one.

We passed Matthew around like a football; everyone holding him and then passing him on—enjoyment for us all. Everyone helped to make this day possible and there was genuine happiness in the mist of the void of Susan still being in the hospital. Susan called on the phone, so we put her on the speaker. Not much anyone could say that could make this experience anything but painful to Susan. "Oh he is cute!" "He is enjoying himself." "He is so alert and laughing." I am not sure how much more Susan wanted to hear or could tolerate hearing. I told her I would be downtown to be with her as soon as I could.

November 22 - Sunday: 6:50 a.m.

I didn't have time to finish the story of Matthew's homecoming.

The party was nice. Everyone pitched in and helped. Everyone had pictures taken with Matthew and he was really accepting of being bounced around.

I called Susan about 5:00 p.m., as the welcome home party for Matthew was ending, and told her I was on my way. My mom, sister and daughter would remain to take care of him. The ride downtown was fairly quick. Viola and Otto, Susan's parents, plus Christian, Susan's nephew, were still at the hospital. They had left Matthew's party early to be with Susan on what was an extremely difficult day. She knows he has gone home and she hasn't. What else she comprehends is unclear. What else is there to know? This is enough! How much more can anyone take? Soon after I arrived (like we were on shifts) they left and I prepared dinner. I had brought sandwiches and a piece of Matthew's cake. We just started to eat when she had to use the bedside commode.

I called the nurse (an older lady about 55) and she came in and I stepped out, Susan was helped onto it. Without a doubt this is the worst experience for her or anyone else. Not being able to take care of her personal hygiene is degrading. Even if everything goes well, the nurse is helpful, privacy is respected, she can feel clean, it still is a degrading experience.

The nurse said to call her when Susan was finished and she'd help her back to bed. After about five minutes, the nurse returned. I stayed outside and then I heard her yell:

"I'm falling." There was a thud; I rushed in and realized Susan must have hit her head on the base of the food tray. She was lying on her side on the floor. The nurse couldn't pick her up and Susan was crying.

I tried to calm her as I picked her up. There was shit on the floor, her hospital gown, herself, and the bed. She was humiliated and started sobbing. "I don't want you to see me like this." That's all she could say, over and over, "I don't want you to see me like this."

"I know you don't, but I don't care. Nothing changed for me. I love you. Let's get you back in bed and cleaned up. We can talk about what I should see later."

This, on top of Matthew leaving, did her in. You could see the pain in her face—the loss of privacy—the total dependency—the fear she would never be herself or get her independence back. Susan had become Matthew—very dependent on others. That fact was killing her and crushing her spirit.

Another nurse arrived and began to help. We changed the bed sheets, her gown, got her cleaned up and back together. The physical trauma is one thing, the blow to self worth is hard to calculate, but you know it's there.

I told her I understood she didn't want me to see her like that—"neither did I". I joked. But it happened and it's over. I sympathized with her, but I had to help. I reassured her that "'til the end of time," it was she and I with Matthew.

"We will get our life back—you will be Susan again—that is the goal. That's what we will achieve—nothing less. You have to believe!" This would become our mantra. A mantra she had to believe wholeheartedly. It is hard to believe when the situation is bleak and unbelievable. Knowing Susan, though, she will find a way to believe. In spite of the darkness she will focus on the one ray of light that is left.

Eventually everything settled down. "At least the food wasn't ruined," I said, attempting another joke. "Well if it didn't taste like shit before it probably does now," she responded. Susan and I learned quickly that jokes and laughter are essential to our survival. Without humor, the pain was overwhelming, overbearing, all-consuming. Without laughter the weight of the pain would crush you. Susan was back. Pissed and caustic – what a great combination.

I set up the tray with the sandwich and the welcome home cake, and we talked about the day, as she picked at both. Melinda called and that helped. I left about 9:00 p.m. I asked, "Do you want to make sure you're clean?" She did. So I wet some cloths and a towel and Susan cleaned up again—just to be sure.

To have lost the basics represents the gap between where you are and where you want to be. Losing the basics can make you expect less. Like "I just want to take care of myself"—"please let me walk"—while these phrases are vital, they represent a step down from her life before the stroke—shopping, making love, driving, working, etc.

When there is nothing—anything is better. But just anything won't do, if you want your life and more back. We both know that. That is the spirit which will drive her.

November 23 - Monday: 8:10 a.m.

I stayed up after Matthew's 6:30 a.m. feeding. He was a nighthawk—up from 7:10 p.m. until 11:30 p.m. He had gas and maybe a cold. He slept from 11:30 p.m. until 2:30 a.m.; 4:30 a.m. until 6:30 a.m. Now he is back sleeping. When he gets up at 9:00 a.m., he will have a bath, a change of clothes and get ready for a new day. He'll take the bottle and stay up for awhile before taking a nap.

Grandma did well. Once you have cared for a baby you don't forget what to do. Once you get the hang of it, it is like you have done this all your life. We were both up at the two early morning feedings. We are all set to get him going for his bath. We have to plan ahead and be prepared.

I know Susan is wondering how she is going to do this. I have two hands and need four more, plus an extra set of eyes, etc. Her doing anything is better than what we have now, so we'll take it as it comes. I'm sure some accommodations, adaptations, short cuts can be thought of which will allow her to be involved in his care. These will happen as we figure out what needs to be done.

Dora, my former secretary, is visiting today. She has graciously offered to help my mother take care of Matthew. I will show her the ropes. Alisa and Grandma are feeding Matthew. Dora has agreed to come over to our home each day to help my mom. Grandma did well but we all know the demands of a child, a newborn, can seem overwhelming. Thank goodness for Dora.

Chapter 5

WHAT IS POSSIBLE?

"For myself, I am an optimist – it does not seem to be much use in being anything else."

- Winston Churchill

November 25 - Wednesday: 6:40 a.m.

I know I say this all the time, but there is no time. Every time you think there is a moment, there is something else to do. I would like to write every day, but when to fit it in is the question.

A number of things have happened:

Susan moved to rehab on Tuesday. She was very disappointed that it didn't happen Monday, but at least she moved. She is making real progress. She can bend her left arm at the elbow and close her fingers (can't open them yet, but that will come). She is beginning to wonder just how much real control she has in closing her hand. Does she have any ability to open it?

Dora arrived today to help my Mom. This will give my Mother a second pair of hands. How Mother keeps up her pace at her age is incredible. But she and Dora are of the old school— work, work, and more work. Expect nothing and you won't be disappointed.

I took Matthew to the pediatrician. Talk about being overwhelmed with getting organized, bathed, and dressed, etc., only to undress him when I got there. He is doing well—gaining weight and appears to be fine.

Matthew had an "all-nighter" on Monday. He didn't sleep for 25 hours, maybe longer (or maybe I didn't sleep for 25 hours), who knows! He had gas and needs to burp more. Also, didn't shit all day. Well, last night (Tuesday evening) he had an atomic shit that made up for everything.

I have tried to keep working. I find it impossible to concentrate on work. I will try and extend my work hours next week and see how it goes. So far, I've been able to juggle things. I go in early, leave at lunch time and spend the afternoon with Susan; have an early dinner with her and then head home to see what awaits me.

I paid some bills this morning. Things are going to start to pile up soon. I hope to get some money from somewhere. Note: the word is "hope."

I've noticed that I have to try and schedule better. I stayed too long at work today and then found myself in a time bind with other demands. So far, I haven't lost my mind—at least I don't think so.

Rehab is a grim place. Susan is in a ward of four beds, about as low as it goes. She arrived yesterday. We are hoping they move her today into a semi-private room, so she can have some privacy and "unpack." It was either take the first bed at rehab or wait for a private room. At the time, the first bed seemed a great idea until you are one of four in a four-bed ward and realize how bad a decision it was.

The first impression of the four-bed unit was bleak, overcrowded, lacking in personal space and privacy. Everyone can hear what you are saying. Such an environment is extremely depressing – and I can leave. Staying and living there is another matter.

Susan had a bladder infection so when the nurse came in Susan said she was having difficulty urinating due to the infection. "That's great! I can see that this is going to be a hell of a night," said the nurse. Just the kind of remark to dash any positive thoughts. I can't imagine the nurse coming quickly when Susan needs to go to the bathroom. I can't imagine Susan wanting to ask for assistance given this nurse's attitude. If it were me, I'd piss in bed and after a few sheet changes maybe attitudes would change or I'd have a red ass because no one ever came to change the sheets.

All the initial assessments by her doctor and the other health care professionals are encouraging. Susan has movement in her left leg and arm and can do more things than the doctor initially expected. Again, the key issue is the comparison point— more than they expected, but nowhere near what she was able to do before. The goal is to narrow this gap. More importantly, the goal is to be who you were. One has to raise the expectation bar, not lower it.

I talked with Susan on the phone and she restated her position that she did not want to be a "burden." "Where have you heard that phrase, don't want to be a burden?" I asked. I told her not to use that word again. She will pull her own weight sooner or later as I jokingly said, "I'm tired of all the household responsibilities. Your vacation will have to end soon."

While at rehab, Susan can go out for walks, dinner in the cafeteria, and have home visits. When all this can start depends on her health and her physical progress. But the sooner one can do these activities the better one feels.

The uncertainty of the future and what functioning/capabilities will return is the mental and emotional weight that hangs over her head (and mine) every waking moment. It is <u>the</u> thought, <u>the</u> only thought. So you try and minimize this uncertain future by noting what new abilities have been attained. Doing small things represents progress. A word, a phrase, "I'm really happy with Susan's progress" says her doctor. Well to be honest, I don't really care how happy the doctor is. How happy is Susan? She is the only judge that counts. Whatever anyone else thinks is beside the point. She sets the goal and only she can determine if it is achieved.

Everything we talk about, plan and hope for, and anticipate is always clouded by this uncertainty. So, when Susan remarks, "I hope I will get better," there is this cloud of doubt. "Will it happen—how much will I get back? What kind of life will I have?" Obviously more questions, far more questions, than answers.

I have been trying to reach her by phone all day today with no success. Turns out she was in a variety of physical, occupational and speech therapy evaluation sessions most of the day. As she puts it, "They're trying to figure out what there is left to work with."

When I finally reached her, she didn't sound happy. Confronting her limitations brings reality home quickly.

"The social worker told me to apply for a handicap license plate. I asked "why?" She told me because I am disabled and will need it. I've never thought of myself as disabled or handicapped, but I guess it is time. It's true. There is no denying this reality. I can't walk—do anything—take care of myself—they're right. I am disabled."

"Physically challenged—temporarily—that is the situation. Don't let anyone set limitations for

you. It's too early—you have to believe and work at
getting back who you are and what you were—then
you can be whatever there is to be." I said.

This is the struggle—confronting limitations
at every turn makes it difficult to see beyond the
moment. The future is too difficult to envision given
the immediacy of the present. The present prevents a
hopeful view of the future. Uncertainty as to what
level of functioning will return is the overwhelming
reality. Uncertainty is the future! Since no one seems
to know, it makes sense to aim high – shoot for the
stars – why? Why not?!

Time frames conjure up memories and
hopes. The way things were before the stroke is the
only point of comparison. Can she - and we - ever be
like we were?

Thanksgiving, November 26 1992 - Thursday

I'm thankful for Susan being alive and able to move ahead;
for Matthew being healthy and for us as a family. It's a great
Thanksgiving to have a second chance at life.

My sister and Mother bought and prepared Thanksgiving
dinner. It was very hectic and busy getting the home ready in time
for the feast.

I talked with Susan a few times in the morning. She was
depressed about the day—the place—the situation. Who can
blame her? Who would be happy institutionalized?
Institutionalized on a holiday yet!

In spite of the day, and the great meal, my thoughts are
with Susan. I'm sure the same is true for her. I'd be extremely
thankful if she were home.

Her mother and dad, Carole and Jim, Melinda, and the
rest of the family, all visited Susan throughout the day. It kept her
going and active because it's a slow day at the hospital. Amy and I
will take the full turkey meal with all the trimmings and Matthew
to visit later in the day.

The coordination and time it takes to get organized is unbelievable. I had to bring clothes for her, food for her, Matthew (and his stuff), plus the meal. I don't know how people do all this by themselves, but I'm learning.

I finally got going about 4:00 p.m. It didn't take long to get there. We parked right in front and went in to see her. Carole and Jim were there. Susan was ecstatic to see Matthew; she broke down crying. The pain of seeing him, but not being able to care for him is overwhelming. It is a constant source of heartache for Susan.

Renee, her nurse, is very nice. She arranged for a family room, so we could visit and have dinner as a family. This was a great idea, because it was out of the way and gave us some privacy.

It is hard to see Susan struggle with practically everything. If she is holding Matthew and starts to cry, she can't wipe her tears or blow her nose. Either I help her or she has to give up Matthew. It seems simple enough, yet who do you know that has to do things this way? That's the point. No one!

If she holds Matthew, she can't touch him because the left arm isn't up-to-speed. I have to hold him close to her so she can touch him. She hasn't been able to see him in his crib, wash him, and change him— nothing. Detached, passive, looking in – whatever phrase one likes it is all the same. Susan is unable, physically, to be part of his life right now. We will have to devise ways for her to be Mom – to feel like his Mom.

We had a good visit, but it was depressing. Susan looked so sad. She could hardly talk. She was happy to see Matthew, but her face reflectsed pain, not joy.

Time does go quickly when you don't want it to. After an hour or so we were headed back to her room to organize and put away her clothes. We had to get an "outfit" picked out for tomorrow. "Outfit" is everything one is going to wear in a day all piled high or stacked so it can be accessed easily. No time to search and decide what to wear. Susan can't do either right now – so "outfits" are the way to go. Five stacks of clothes, one for each day of the week. Here I am trying to organize socks, underwear, bras, and pants, to get her ready for the next day. Take home her dirty clothes, clean up her area, get her tray organized—all things that show her limitations. Clothes, a favorite of hers, are now a challenge. What isn't a challenge? Simple clothes, sweats, t-shirts. No buttons, belts, or ties. Not exactly what she would choose to wear.

Leaving that evening with Matthew was difficult. It's like we just arrived and now we have to head home so the rest of the family can see Matthew. Besides, there is nowhere to really visit in the present room set up. The family visiting room is a converted office, but it is quiet and away from the hospital room, so that is better than anything else.

November 27 - Friday: 7:20 a.m.

Matthew cooperated! I stayed up later than usual so he could get his 11:30 feeding—then he slept right through until 5:10 a.m. He did his part to give us all a rest.

I talked with Susan earlier this morning, and she sounded tired! She said she slept well; that means she didn't stay awake all night. She was going to get ready for physical therapy and other rehab activities—hope it is a good day for her.

Speaking of rehab – the facility has a "unique" way of letting the patient know the schedule of activities for the day. The schedule is taped to the <u>back</u> of the wheelchair so staff can easily see it. The schedule looks like a price tag ticket – in fact the first time I saw the tag, I assumed the wheelchair was new and the patient was trying it on for size.

Patients don't have a copy they can see or hold – just the copy on the back of the chair. Susan would say she was startled all day long by individuals coming up from behind and pushing her off to the next session. No, "How are you?" or "I'm Tom and I have come to take you to occupational therapy or wherever." None of that. "Just out of the blue someone pushing your wheelchair to the next appointment that only they knew," she continued.

In fact the more I think about the "schedule tag" and the "pushers" (support staff who move the patients to their appointments) the more insensitive and inhumane I think this experience is. The patient has neither input nor any participation

71

in this scheduling – transportation experience. It is just done to him/her. So much for Rehab's number 1 ranking as the "best rehab facility" in the United States. I am sure if any patients had been solicited for their opinion, the #1 ranking might be in jeopardy. However, if this facility is ranked #1, I certainly would not want to be in a lower-ranked center.

The other facet of this patient movement is that all those who are going somewhere are lined up outside their hospital rooms, like a staggered start at a car race event. When an appointment is completed the person is pushed out into the hall (with others) lined up and waits to be moved again. Sort of like rolling starts after each session. Then the chairs are lined up at the elevators for what is called "boarding." Chairs are pushed in facing the back wall which is all the patient sees. Anyone standing (meaning staff) are facing forward. Obviously, an inhumane experience.

Clearly, this works for the rehab staff. But I am not sure anyone has thought to ask the patients if it "works" for them.

My Mom left with Betty to go into the city. My Mom lives in Chicago, and Susan and I live in a suburb. My Mom will get her hair done, check the mail, etc. It's a good idea to take a break; she'll return later. It is a responsibility to take care of Matthew and I can see it is taking a toll on her.

So it's Matthew and me (plus Hans – the dog) alone in the house. I am solely responsible (a scary thought) for Matthew's care. I have picked up and started wash, putting away the dinner dishes, etc. My sisters have been doing the bulk of the housework— cooking and cleaning, etc. Eventually this has to end and it is one more thing to fit in.

I'm going to the "Y" this morning to get my stuff and go see the guys at the annual post Turkey Day Bash. Matthew will stay home with Nana (the name my Mother prefers). I don't know when, or if, I will ever return to the "Y." I will say thanks for their thoughts and the flowers they sent; then I will go to the grocery store and then back home. I have to figure out who is going to watch Matthew later in the day so I can visit Susan. I will work on that later.

I went to see Susan in the late afternoon. Traffic on the expressway was light due to the holiday, but the shoppers were out in full force. Luck was with me. I found a parking spot on the street.

Rehab is truly a "cuckoo's nest"—all sizes, shapes and impairments. Susan said going out to the "group feed" for morning and afternoon meals is a real experience. The "group feed" happens at every meal. All meals are to be eaten in the group room at whatever table they put you at. Staff members never ask, "Where would you like to sit?" Everyone is staring at you, staring at the wall, just looking into space. If you complain, or in anyway show your displeasure with this arrangement, the nurses will be sure to make you "the last one to go back" to your room. So Susan sits for 85 minutes because she can't get back to her room on her own. There are no choices; no compassion. The "food," having been cooked and placed in steam carts for over an hour before arriving on the floor, is barely edible. After five minutes of picking at the plate of food Susan only has 80 minutes to kill. It gives her too much time to reflect.

The living arrangement is very depressing. Hard to determine whether the "group feed" or the "four in the ward" is the worse of the worst. Depressing is the defining word. Since four are in the ward room, there is a rotation of showers. No one is able to shower every day. No real privacy. Someone can be using the bathroom while another patient showers. Only a shower curtain – plastic at that - separating them. Isn't this the way you want to spend your time? Is this how you want to live? Would any nurse or physician like to be treated this way? I don't think they would, yet it is a standard practice for patients.

Susan looks depressed and beaten down. Her physical posture, her hair, the downward cast to her eyes doesn't do justice to the life and vitality she had. She finally received a wheelchair that fits her. She also received a backpack to put stuff in rather then carry it all day. At night the staff line-up the patients' wheelchairs outside their rooms. Susan was very worried that her wheelchair would be taken during the night. That it would not be there in the morning. I couldn't believe she was worried about where they were putting her chair. But as she pointedly informed me, "You would be worried about the chair if that was all you had or your only way to get around." A point well made.

She continued, "See, that's how bad it is. I'm worried about my wheelchair and knapsack. Who's crazy? That is what rehab can do – make you begin to think about things in ways that can change you."

I said, "Let them take the chair – they will get you another one if it is missing."

"But you don't know, you don't live here," Susan said. She sees herself as living there; I have to get her out of this place as soon as possible to save her mind.

It has only been 5 days since she was transferred from the hospital to rehab. Susan and I had a saying "the road home goes through rehab." Little did we know what a long haul this was going to be. She is just starting her rehab so there is really no way to judge how long it will take or what progress we can expect. At this point it just doesn't feel like she is going to make it through this experience. I know and she knows, that eventually this stay at rehab will end.

When the end is nowhere in sight, it is a very uncertain experience.

November 28 - Saturday: 8:00 a.m.

My Mother gave us a loan of $5,000 to pay bills and cover expenses. I spent an hour and a half going through all the mail and bills over the last month. I will mail them out this morning. Talk about depressing—but I really don't give a shit. I'll either pay them or declare bankruptcy.

We already received a few hospital bills. The first hour working on Matthew cost $1,700, not counting the doctor's bills. Who cares? We'll see what's possible and what's not. Bills are no longer a real priority.

Matthew had a decent night. He went down about 11:30 p.m.; up at 2:00 a.m.; up at 5:15 a.m. He has gas which makes him have cramps. I really have to try and burp him after he eats, otherwise he is very uncomfortable.

Hans was happy. It was Saturday, so we went to the bakery. That's a favorite thing of his to do. We stopped at the bank and bakery. I will do some shopping later.

I talked with Susan. She slept okay, "I really can't wait to get home." Who can blame her? She continued, "Sleep is my only peace; I wake up to this nightmare and each day gets worse. Being fuckin' paralyzed is no picnic." It is the first time I heard her use the word paralyzed when referring to herself.

She was already teary-eyed at 8:00 a.m.
Not a real good way to start the day. She said, "Well
now that I am up, I can begin to live the nightmare.
The bad news is that it doesn't go away—it will
never go away." What do I say to her? What can
anyone say? Words are an empty response to such a
loss. "So what else is new?" I said. "We just have to
keep moving – just get through the next minute,
hour, day or whatever. Vent and move on—
hopelessness will kill the spirit. If you loose hope you
will not survive." Remarks meant for me as well as
her.

I did errands today. I paid the bills with the money mother loaned us. I went grocery shopping, to the cleaners, to the hardware store. You name it and I made the stops.

I tried to give my Mother a break. She tries to do everything but it will wear her out. So I do what I can of the child care, washing, changing, and feeding. She went back to sleep this morning which was a good idea.

Alisa and I took a ride to see Susan this afternoon. My mother and sister, Betty, wanted to shop tonight at Field's. Stores are open late—good time to do shopping. Also, Matthew needed some clothes—like a sweater set.

Therefore, Alisa and I went into the city to see Susan early afternoon. Carole was there, as well as Susan's mother and father. At least the visitors break up the day for her. Her day is made up of waiting for tests, visitors, or for the day to end. Susan had a variety of physical and occupational therapy/speech activities today in her room, which kept her busy. Visitors just give you something to look forward to, otherwise you feel like you're a prisoner. As Susan has reminded me, *"Feel like a prisoner?! You think this is freedom?"*

Susan is struggling with her feelings, limitations and frustrations. The basics, like going to the bathroom, are a monumental task. So now she has a bladder infection which makes her feel like she has to go when she really doesn't. Then you have to call the nurse and go through the federal case of getting out of bed, into the chair, onto the pot, back to the chair, and back to bed—every 25 minutes.

After about two of these "requests for help," she lost it. Who wouldn't? I told her it was okay to have her feelings of anger and disgust, but we'd get beyond it and get our life back. We just have to do what has to be done to get through this nightmare. This lesson we will learn every day, perhaps for the rest of our lives.

She was feeling overheated from all the moving around. I helped her change from a sweatshirt to a T-shirt and even this seemingly simple task is a struggle. To get her sweatshirt off, fix her bra, try to get her T-shirt on: the bad hand in first and then the good, then over the head and straighten it out the collar, even the shoulders. A federal case. Helping can get in the way, so the first rule is to "ask." If the response is "No, I don't need any help." then don't help no matter how long it takes. This lesson needs to be learned quickly. It has taken me far too long to learn it. ASK. Always ASK. If the answer is "no thanks, I can do it" then you have to back off no matter how difficult the struggle is or how long it takes. Speed and ease of task are not important. Being able to do it by oneself is the goal – the only goal. Accomplishing the task is another step closer to independence. Having said that, it is not easy watching Susan struggle with her coat or undoing a button. My tendency is to just jump in and do it for her. Take over for her - she would say. Therefore, ask!

Alisa and I talked in the car about how she and Amy thought they were being deserted when I married Susan. The house, the baby, a whole new family—why need them? In a perverted way, they laughed about the baby having colic or something—to sort of make it hard—rub it in.

Funny how such a tragedy makes you grow up and quickly. How you realize the importance of family and the things you take for granted. A good lesson in life learned the hard way. The girls now realize more than ever the importance in their life of Susan, their mother and me. They also now see Matthew as a brother, rather than as a rival.

Susan has started to talk about the "inmate mentality," institutionalization feelings; how you are trapped wherever you are until the staff brings you back to your room. The patronizing style of some staff who say, "You've been good, so you can go back to your room." As Susan knows too well, "Hope you're never bad— God only knows what would happen or where the staff would take you."

Well it's time to rest. I agree with Susan that sleep is the only time I am at peace. The nightmare returns every morning. I'm closing my eyes as I write. I'm so tired. Enough for today, more tomorrow.

November 29- Sunday: 10:02 a.m.

I was exhausted last night. I went to bed at 9:40 p.m. and left my mom to care for Matthew. I had hoped to get a good start on sleep before the 3:00 or 4:00 a.m. feeding. No such luck.

Matthew fussed a bit and my mom tried to rock him. I got up with him at 11:00 p.m., then again at 2:00 a.m. (when I fell asleep feeding him), up at 4:15 a.m. when I fed him and told my mom to get some sleep. I took Hans out about 5:00 a.m., and then fell asleep on the couch with my jacket on until 8:00 a.m. All-in-all, not too bad. I'm going to have to learn to take naps whenever I can. That is what sleep has become, a series of naps throughout the night.

As the days pass (three weeks yesterday since the stroke), the scope and magnitude of the problem is escalating. Susan is very worried about her left arm and hand (everybody has been cautious about it from the beginning). Her leg is "more alive than this dead arm," as she puts it, "and the left leg really doesn't work that well - so what does that say about the arm?"

The weeks have been bearable for me because of the holidays. Next week, a full work week should be a real challenge. I plan to go in early, come home and help out, and then head to rehab for a couple of hours. Sometimes I'll leave right from work so as to get home earlier to help my mother or do whatever else needs to be done.

I talked with Susan about 8:30 a.m. today. I can hear the despair in her voice.

> *"Another day, what a joke. Here I lie*
> *waiting for someone to show me how to get dressed—*
> *what a joy! I should be dressing Matthew not having*
> *someone dress me! I just can't believe it. Here I am*
> *and there is nothing – absolutely nothing I can do*
> *about it. In fact there is nothing I can do period.*
> *Who am I kidding? I need help with everything!"*

A brutal, frank, and unfortunately honest characterization of her situation.

She continues to express concern about her left arm and hand. Even she is aware of the profound impairment and limitations. You only have two hands and if one doesn't work, how long will the other one last?

> *"I'm really worried about my left arm and*
> *hand. It is no where near as good as the leg, and the*
> *leg isn't great..."*

> *"I know, I know. I think it's too early to*
> *tell, plus the electrical stimulation treatments have to*
> *be tried. Who knows? But we will get back—*
> *somehow, some way, we will make things happen.*
> *The hand will come back in due time."*

I can't imagine the level of fear, apprehension and anxiety she faces, let alone the depression from realizing the present circumstances and the less-than-optimistic forecast. These

78

emotions are enough to blow your mind away—not to mention mess with your focus on recovery. What else are you to think about? At every turn, step, task, you confront a limitation, impairment – more simply, reality hits you in the face all day long. Yet, Susan continues to persevere. Her actions speak volumes about her courage and determination.

I'm feeling more depressed about the situation, the overwhelming nature of these events has not directly impacted me yet, but the lack of sleep and the endless list of chores and activities are taking its toll. When I begin to feel this way, I think about Susan and my concerns pale by comparison.

The overwhelming sense of uncertainty casts a pall over our daily thoughts and activities. The mornings are the worst since the reality confronts you upon awakening. In Susan's case, she is hit with the reality of paralysis and helplessness. In my case, it's the responsibilities of caring for her and Matthew. For Susan and me it is the uncertainty – the absolute uncertainty about everything. The only thing that is certain is that this feeling of uncertainty will be here a while and it may never leave.

Hope is the only refuge from the pain and reality of the daily events. I'm reminded of the statement, "hope is a great breakfast, but a lousy dinner." Hope is nurtured by a faith in a better day (course of events), as well as concrete actions that indicate progress. You need both to sustain it. We need more indicators of progress to keep us moving. Belief is important but there is no substitute for being able to do things. Seeing and feeling progress is critical. It is essential. Sooner or later you have to put up or shut up.

November 30 - Monday: 8:45 a.m.—at the office

I am sorry to keep repeating myself, but there is no time— it is hard to believe that you can go at the pace I am going and continue to fall behind.

Briefly, here's what's been happening:

Susan continues to make slow progress, which is the same as no progress in her mind. Each day, she realizes her severe limitations which reinforce her despair over being unable to regain her old self. Now she is not real sure she likes what the "new self" will be—even though what the "new self" will be is still unclear. We pretend to talk as if there are choices—this is it until it changes and/or improves. The delusion of choices is comforting – at least for now.

She loves when the baby visits. She enjoyed the Sunday get-together. She looks forward to each visit—and hates to see Matthew go. It is extremely difficult for her to find a way to be part of his life, to take care of him. That's the pain—being unable to participate in what she wanted so much.

She is up and down in her spirits. Who wouldn't be?! The psychologist came by and told her she "had a full plate of things to deal with"—what a fuckin' insight. This kind of pat response drives me nuts! "A full plate—fuck him!" she said. I love the clarity of her thinking and how succinctly she can characterize her feelings and make her point.

Matthew has been doing well, although he doesn't "cooperate" at night. Last night, he finally went to bed at 11:00 p.m. and got up at 2:00 a.m., and then got up at 5:15 a.m. I will try more formula to see if that holds him. Also, he has gas— doesn't burp easy—that contributes to things being hard for him.

At night when I go (or try to go) to sleep, I'm so tired that I can't think straight. I find myself sitting in a trance, and holding Matthew who is crying at the top of his lungs. With so many things going on, I tend to lose focus. Let me give you an example.

I was running late at work, so I didn't get home until 2:00 in the afternoon, instead of 1:00 p.m. Dora and my mother were going shopping, but they decided I could take them. We went to four stores in an hour and 45 minutes. I was rushing to get home, so I could head downtown. I made a sandwich to eat in the car.

I backed out of the driveway and thought I looked both ways. As I reached the street, I saw a school bus out of the corner of my eye, slammed on the brakes and just missed backing into a speeding school bus. What a joy that would have been. That event caught my attention real quick. I became oriented to time and place in a hurry.

I'm going to stay home from the hospital today—first day I will miss seeing Susan—and help my mom and Matthew. I will try to take a nap and rest up. It will be difficult not to see Susan today.

I have begun planning our wedding anniversary party for Wednesday. I will have it catered, if I can arrange it. Some special meal will be brought in by a company that does this as a business. I hope it turns into a special day. It is a special day for me and for Susan. It just doesn't seem special given the circumstances.

I have to get on with work. I will stop for now. When I start up again, I'll write some about how you have to think about things and how Susan and I are going about it.

December 1 - Tuesday: 1:50 p.m.

I'm at Rolling Meadows High School waiting to give Amy a ride to the house. She'll stay with Grandma, while I head downtown.

Tomorrow is our second anniversary—a mixed day at best given the uncertain future. Not uncertain about us. We are together until the end of time. Uncertain as to what the future holds. It's a great day because we're together. That is for certain! I called Susan this morning and chatted on the phone. She sounded good, although I had her on the speaker phone and she may not have wanted to say anything with Grandma present. Never thought of that till now—well there's an example of sensitivity.

I went out and bought some cards and a watch for her to have downtown. I'm bringing her wedding band in the ring case. We'll exchange "I do's."

We were going to go out to eat, but it is cold and this would be her "first time out" of the hospital. She may not be ready for such an outing. So, the catered meal inside is what it is. At least we are together.

December 3 - Thursday: 4:50 p.m.

Yesterday was a big day for us - our 2nd wedding anniversary. I arranged for a catering company to bring in two dinners. I arrived downtown early, so we had a chance to visit and talk about the day's activities—something we have a hard time doing due to schedules, visitors, etc.

Carole came by to "paint" Susan's face. It was nice to see her look like her old self. Carole did a great job on her hair and make-up. It was a boost for Susan. It made her feel "with it" and back to her old ways. Dinner was excellent and the family room had been reserved for our use. I set the table and prepared the drinks – two Diet Cokes. We really enjoyed ourselves. It was perfect. Next year, we will look back at the 2nd anniversary as a bad memory. At least that is our fervent prayer.

My Mother and Amy had a tough time with Matthew— it's a long day with lots of responsibilities. Plus, it's been two weeks without a break. My mom is worn-out. Who wouldn't be? She tried to say in a nice way that I can't keep going down to the hospital every day. "You'll drop dead," was her subtle comment. I agreed, but until I drop dead, I'll keep going.

The bind is when do I: take care of Matthew; visit Susan; work. There is not enough of me to go around. Susan and I talked about this problem of visiting and the schedule, so it's not news to us. For me, not seeing her each day is worse than being tired. I am glad my mother said what she did, because she is right, nevertheless, this is the schedule.

It is hard not being with Susan. I know she is lonely and afraid and wants my assurance that she is important in my life. Well you can say that and/or show it. I've tried to do both and I am running out of gas. If either one of us (Mother or I) got sick or came down with the flu, then the house of cards would collapse.

My Mother is having her hair done tonight. At least she can get out for a while. Dora has been a blessing—I am not sure my mother could go day after day without the help of Dora.

Work is picking up. I am trying to focus on our research and related projects to get things going again. I put in six hours at the office, then leave and do work at home or read on the train.

Susan and I have been talking about retaining legal representation because of the mishandling of Susan's care by Dr. Toig, her OB/Gyn. I don't want to be distracted by this because the focus is on Susan and her rehabilitation, that's the #1 priority. Nevertheless, this is a matter that needs and deserves attention.

The issue of malpractice was raised by both of her physicians. In essence, their question to me was "what went wrong?" I certainly didn't have an answer, but the way they raised the question implied that something did go wrong. If proper care was provided, Susan would not be in this situation. The hypertension should have been treated. The stroke was preventable. Not a comforting thought. If someone had done their job everything would have been ok. Instead, well you knowÖ

"A third-year medical student would know what to do – obviously the doctors/residents must not have known because the stroke occurred," to quote one of Susan's physicians.

I will explore this issue and I am sure talk more about it as time passes.

It is nice to be at home alone. All the calls, and even my Mom always being around, doesn't allow for any quiet time. Don't get me wrong, without Dora and Mom, I'd collapse. It's just that quiet is nice. No questions. Just silence.

Susan sounded real positive on the phone. Rehab is demanding work and she works hard everyday. The ophthalmologist said her chances of regaining eyesight in both eyes (especially the left) are excellent. That's what you want to hear and believe! It's nice that our beliefs can be confirmed once in a while by some outside source.

December 4 - Friday: 8:10 p.m.

Taking the train into the city to see Susan is a break from driving. I do it occasionally. Currently, I am on the train waiting for it to pull out of the station and head home. I took the train because of Friday night/Christmas traffic, but there was none. Everyone stayed in the city for Christmas parties.

So what's been happening? This is a question I frequently ask myself just to see if I can recall all that is happening.

Susan has an eight-hour pass scheduled for Sunday. Unbelievable that she can get out and spend time at home. That's the best news she has had, we all have had, in a long time.

Matthew has been real good. I gave him the "gas medication" and that seems to help. Betty, my sister, is staying overnight so Mom and I should get a good night's sleep—we'll see.

They are going to go shopping tomorrow. I'll take Matthew downtown and then it'll be just the two of us for the night and the next day. There shouldn't be any problem, just responsibilities.

When we are visiting, Susan can help in caring for him. That will be real good for her and all of us. She needs to do things for him to believe and feel like his Mom.

I continue to get advice and suggestions that we have, or will have, a major lawsuit pending. From everything we hear, we have a solid case/basis for such an action. So what if you do, you still may not have yourself back, or whole. We will have to see what happens over time.

Work has been going okay—good meeting today. Various projects are moving forward and everyone has assigned tasks. It is good to get back doing that. I still can't really get into it, but I will continue to try to work in order to get back to normal. However, getting back to normal at home is a hope that is fading fast. Things are so different and the future, who am I kidding, tomorrow is not really knowable. I really don't think "we will get back" – so it's the unknown future that lies ahead. The future will unfold as we go, so there is no reason to worry about it. This is easier said than done.

But I do often wonder what the future holds. I guess it's normal to be apprehensive about the future, but I am also optimistic that things will work out. They always have seemed to in the past—so why should things change now? Call me Mr. Optimistic! Is there really any other choice?

Susan is looking like her old self. She has made great strides, but there is still much progress to make. I helped her to the bathroom tonight before I left. I never would have imagined doing that, let alone her allowing me to, yet it's okay because that's what it is now and will have to be until that changes.

I picked up the Christmas wreaths today on the way home. I hung them up outside and will get the floodlight going so the home looks like Christmas. I will try and get a tree, so it can go up next week. That way the house will start to look like the holidays. Holidays are important to Susan. She always has the appropriate displays ready to mark the special holidays.

I have received all the disability/insurance forms to complete for the feds; for work; and for the private insurance carrier. I hope these applications are reviewed and approved quickly so that some financial assistance will be available.

I have to think about a different car. Do I dare mention a van? I will sell the Hans-mobile, our small, two-door Honda Civic that our dog always accompanies us in as we do errands on the weekend. Our four-door Honda does not have the room we will need for a wheelchair and/or an electric scooter. I will have to see what I can work out.

I was very emotional today when I discussed with Susan the family next door to her at rehab who had to make the difficult—almost incomprehensible—decision to remove a 36-year-old woman from a respirator. She had suffered a stroke the Friday of Matthew's birth. The stroke occurred during childbirth and she was now in a vegetative state. The doctors did not give her husband any hope for a recovery. There was no brain wave activity. He decided to disconnect her life support since she was already brain dead. In talking with Susan, I just broke down. I'm so glad I didn't have to do that. Talking about that possibility was bad enough. No one ever plans to talk about such life and death decisions with anyone. To be presented with the possibility of your spouse dying is unfathomable. To actually have to make a decision is.

December 5 - Saturday: 6:10 p.m. (1 month post surgery)
It is hard to believe a month has passed. What an unbelievable month! I wonder how long we can keep this up. Guess the answer is simple: as long as it takes. There are decisions, expectations, plans, and uncertainties, more uncertainties than anything. Undoubtedly there are more unknowns to come. What lies ahead, I don't know. I just know with certainty that uncertainty lies ahead and we will confront it together.

Betty stayed overnight, which is not real easy for her. Matthew didn't cooperate and Betty has to learn some of the tricks. She was up with him at 1:15 a.m. and 5:10 a.m. Quite a schedule.

Mother said for the first time that she "feels old." That's how all of this has affected her. Her sleep, schedule, eating and activities are all off—plus, she is working hard taking care of Matthew. She is taking Saturday off—maybe Sunday. I want her to go home for a few days and sleep in her own bed. I hope she does it.

I took Matthew and his supplies downtown to see Susan. It is quite a production to get him, his stuff, and me organized and coordinated. I was downtown early (10:30 a.m., not 11:00 a.m.). Susan enjoyed the day. She was pacing (in the wheelchair) by the elevator. She was very anxious to see us.

The occupational therapist tried to help Susan do some things with Matthew. The disability becomes real when you try to do things or happen to remember that you can't. It's this concrete confrontation with reality that is hard to take. It also jolts you into the real world between the past and hope for the future. This is the way things are now! Nothing can be done about it except to continue to work hard at regaining functions.

The "here and now" is becoming increasingly real and terrifying; it confronts us at every turn with what we don't have and are not quite sure of what we do have. Who cares about what might or might not happen when now you can't walk, go to the bathroom unaided, use your left hand, etc? The moment becomes the only reality that counts.

It was difficult for Susan to try and take care of Matthew. She can do some things, but only with help and assistance. That's fine—for now—if more abilities develop, then all the better. However, it is sort of crazy to try and suggest she can do things for him that she can't for herself. She knows it—so why try stupid exercises like scooping him with one hand. Where do you go if you get him picked up with one hand? She can't walk—so what is the point? I'm not sure rehab understands the full reality of the situation.

86

Susan lost a month of parenting that I have experienced with Matthew. Practice will be helpful for her and her sense of ability. It was good for me to have a chance to get comfortable with him. It takes time and she will figure out what she can do with and for him.

There are so many things to carry and do before we can go anywhere —the baby, the bag, the coat, food tray—everything she needs or wants requires assistance. It is very frustrating for Susan. Today was the first time she actually fed him. It was painful to watch her struggle. There is a sadness in her look and eyes, her shoulders are stooped and rounded, her hair has to be cut—these physical attributes make her look extremely downcast. This image is difficult to reconcile with the bright, forward-moving career woman. This is not her and she knows it. The challenge is to regain herself; who she was and is from the realties of the present situation.

My sister Bobbi and her husband, Tony, paid Susan a visit. We overlapped a bit and Tony helped me to the car. There are many things to carry and too few hands.

Matthew was good on the ride up and back. When I got home, Amy, Betty and my mother appeared. They helped straighten things up, fed Matthew, while I unpacked and got things put away.

They left at 5:00 p.m. I'm on my own tonight. I started the wash and fixed up the beds. Now I'm doing clothes, plus dishes, then his clothes. Whoever said there is no time, you simply let this and that go until it has to be done, was right. You can only do what you can do. Each day you realize how far behind you are – and each day adds to the sense that more and more is not getting done.

I'm going to take a nap, while Matthew is napping. That way we can be on the same page when he awakes. With any luck, he'll be good and I'll get some sleep.

Susan's mother and dad are making dinner and going to come over tomorrow when Susan is home on an 8 hour pass. I hope this doesn't turn into a zoo with a stream of traffic. We'll see.

It is lonely and quiet in the house. Amy took the car tonight. So it's Matthew and me (plus Hans). While he sleeps, you wait for him to get up and repeat the cycle of changing, feeding, and caring. You simply don't know when this will happen again. So your free time (as if there is such a thing) is consumed waiting to start again. That changes as you get more comfortable. Baby or no baby, life goes on. He fits in, you fit in and a new pattern emerges.

It would just be a hell of a lot easier if Susan were here and we could struggle together at this. But her struggle is critical because what she can or can't do will be with us forever. Keep working, dear!

December 6 - Sunday: 7:30 a.m.

Matthew had an easy night. He was up twice at 1:15 a.m. and 5:30 a.m. He stayed up a bit, then went back to sleep. Relatively speaking, this would be a great pattern. He is sleeping a little longer between feedings and he is taking more formula.

I stayed up at 5:30 a.m., so I could get the house together and do wash, bottles, etc. He has cooperated, so everything is done and I've even showered. I am waiting for my mother and sister to come over, so I can leave to get Susan.

Big, big day! After over a month (November 3 - December 7) in the hospital, she will be going outside and home for the first time. Feelings and anticipation are extremely high—emotions will probably be out of control—we can handle that.

I hope the day is quiet, happy and restful. Susan's Mom insisted on cooking and bringing food. I didn't like the idea, but we'll let her do it and see what happens. While I expect some visitors, I don't want a ton of people coming and going. Susan needs rest and a chance to enjoy herself and get reacquainted with our home, the baby, and all that has been happening.

I talked with her already (she was up at 4:00 a.m.). She is very anxious and excited. Of all days, today they are predicting 2-4 inches of snow. Who cares! As long as we can get home, we'll be fine. If we can't make it back due to the weather that will be even better.

December 8 - Tuesday: 7:15 a.m.

I hate to start off by talking about time, but there is none—enough said.

Let's go back to Sunday, December 6th, the first home visit.

Carole, her niece who lives in downtown Chicago, had come over to rehab to help Susan with her hair and makeup. Susan looked smashing when I arrived. "Where were you?" she said. It was 9:45 a.m. and I was running a little late.

Excited is not the word to explain her look and feelings. It was wow—let's get out of here. We were in such a hurry that we didn't have the discharge papers or her take-home medications as we headed for the car. Carole, who was still with us, had to go back and get them.

Finally, we got organized in the hall. She had to put on her coat which was not easy when one of her hands was not working. We finally figured out how to do that by having her stand and put the bad arm in first. Then the good arm, making sure the "bad arm" was all the way through before pulling the coat up and zipping it. No more zippers – buttons forever. I am sure we will figure out how best to do this and a host of other things. Trial and error will have to do for now.

The car transfer (getting her from the chair to the car and back) worked well. We sort of know how to do this. The wheelchair is a hassle; it is a loaner from the Rehabilitation Institute of Chicago (RIC) and one of the foot rests is broken, so it really didn't help support her leg as she sat in the chair. Also, the wheelchair is quite heavy and bulky. No simple task to lift the chair into the back seat. I was going to put it into the trunk, but I had too much junk in it for the chair to fit. I hope the chair that is ordered for her will be much better than this loaner.

"It feels strange to be out—see normal people. Everyone I see at RIC has a chair or something. To see real people is funny. I almost forgot what people looked like," she said. "Nice to see the city and the shops, lights, and just to get out of rehab is great."

As we drove home, I asked her how she felt. "A little dizzy, like things are moving too fast for me. But, if I look straight ahead, I'm okay. I don't think my head has come back together yet."

The ride was very emotionally draining. It had been more than one month since the stroke and much was lost while she was away from home. We missed Thanksgiving, our anniversary, and we're right into Christmas without any real transition. Also, there is this heightened anticipation of being home and seeing Matthew and the dog. Most important, she has missed being a Mom and doing what Mom's do.

Home looked real great to her as we pulled up. The plan was to get her in the chair and let the dog, Hans, come out to see her. I assumed he'd be real excited and there was more room outside to jump around and greet "Mommy," than to have the excitement in the house.

We pulled up, I helped her out and into the wheelchair, and then brought out Hans. He was very excited to see "Mommy," but knew something was very wrong. He sniffed her bad leg as if to say he knew. He sniffed and licked her left hand; tried to move it with his head. He barked at the wheelchair. He didn't like it or her in it. Clearly Hans knew "Mommy" was different and he continued to lick her hand and push her arm with his head as if to say "get working again."

Betty came out to help. I got Susan situated and opened the door to roll her into the house. Being home and being able to comprehend this experience made me realize the profound impact this event has had on our lives.

Clearly the house, built in the 50's, is not set up to be handicap accessible. To begin with, there are stairs that have to be negotiated to enter the house. The doorways are narrow and the wheelchair cannot fit through the door opening into the bathroom. Rugs make pushing the wheelchair more difficult.

Regardless of these first impressions, Susan was grateful to get home, sit down, and do nothing but take in and savor this experience. Relatives and friends were over, wanting to say "Welcome home Susan." Another milestone had been reached. She was home – even if it was only for a brief 8 hour stay. It was a start.

Susan was told by her physician at rehab to buy a wheelchair; she'd need one. "There is little hope that Susan will walk. I'm still optimistic that she'll walk. But she has to be prepared for the reality that she may never walk again." That's the news delivered by her rehab physician at 8:00 a.m. today. I learned of this devastating pronouncement when I stopped by for lunch with Susan after the business meeting I had attended downtown. Devastated is a mild characterization of her feelings, mine included. Shock, disbelief, outrage, anger, denial—add your own adjective to describe my feelings and it is not even close.

These are the feelings I felt and I'm sure Susan was having her own set of feelings at another level. We are talking about Susan, not me. I'm not sure what emotions one should have or how one can keep them all straight when you are told you will not walk again – conveyed bright and early at 8:00 a.m.

This news follows on the proposed discharge date of January 5, 1993. We had hoped – knowing the likelihood was low – but were hopeful nevertheless, of a before-Christmas discharge date. No luck. Speaking of luck, nothing has gone our way since the bleed. In spite of being grateful that there were no post-surgical complications (at least none that we knew of), etc., everything that could go wrong has and continues to go wrong.

I spent 45 minutes with Susan until Beth, one of Susan's best friends, came by to visit before Susan's 1:30 p.m. OT appointment. I told Susan I'd contact her doctor (the physician who broke this news) to see what I could find out. We want to know what "I'm still optimistic" means—a snowball's chance in hell or some decent odds? It is important to know this.

I'm overwhelmed by this news and the prospects for the future. I have to find some full-time help for Matthew, Susan, Hans, the home, etc. Susan needs full-time care herself—that's debilitating to one's mind and spirit. As she said, "I thought, just get me home. Well now I'm home for the visit and, so what—I can't do anything or care for myself. What's the sense of it all?" The joy of seeing and being home wore off quickly.

Home is bittersweet—better than the hospital, but you're really no better off. So all that happened was that Susan changed

locations. No real change in skills or abilities. That's the bind—
and it is difficult to accept. In fact, home presents a host of new
obstacles; maybe I should be positive and say challenges. Hallways
are narrow; the chair won't fit through doorway openings. There is
carpeting that makes it hard to roll the chair (no need to list all of
them, there isn't time or enough paper).

So you hope in a vacuum of hopelessness because of the
doubt over how much functioning and independence will or will
not return (the use of her leg/arm). It's an emotionally draining,
spirit-sapping feeling. The more you deny the reality, the less
prepared you are for the everyday realities you'll confront as a
person with a disability. So the plan is to meet – and defeat – these
challenges head on.

The more you "accept" the reality, the "less hope" you
have for the future. Either position is difficult. Living in both is
impossible. Somehow we will figure out a strategy and move
forward.

In any event, one undeniable truth is abundantly clear, the
way things were will never be again. What remains to be answered
is what the will future be. To that question, no one knows the
answer. She, me, we are changed forever!

December 9 - Wednesday: 7:30 p.m.

I talked with Susan early (6:50 a.m.) She sounded upbeat
and positive -very willing to get on with it. To tell you the truth,
her spirit made me feel better. She is **determined** to do whatever it
takes to regain her life. Being sad or depressed or fed-up with
"everything" are momentary flair-ups that let off steam which
allows her to move forward. I don't know how she is able to do
this but I am very grateful that she can find the will to do so.

This sense of determination is palpable. It is a reservoir of
strength that she has and I can draw upon. Determination cuts
through obstacles better than anything else. Having set the goal the
task is to achieve it any way we can.

I slept fairly well. I talked with Susan's nurses (Renee and
Joanna). It's important to stress that the nurses are everything.
Without them, you're helpless. They (the nurses) can make an

intolerable situation bearable or they can make hell seem like a nice place.

Susan and I talked about remaining positive, moving ahead, and seeing the wheelchair as a minor detour or setback. She has to use it to help herself, but Susan doesn't want it as a permanent part of her life. It's something we will put up with until it is no longer needed.

I told her, "I love you," like the song, "till the end of time." I mean it and want her to keep hearing it. She can have no doubts over where we stand—it's together, forever!

After we talked, I called her back to tell her, "Love ya— have a good day—work hard and focus on what you have to do for yourself."

I can't believe how many bad breaks can occur in this mess. The jolt of not being able to walk is hard to imagine. If you think about it, all sorts of crazy thoughts run through your mind. For instance:

The home—it won't work. Remodel or sell? Neither one is feasible.

What kind of chair—electric? Can you lift an electric cart into the trunk of the car? Would it fit? What does it cost?

Do we need a van?

Total care. Do I have to make arrangements for total care? Susan will need help—for how long, who knows, let alone Matthew. How much help with what is unclear.

I can't leave them alone for any length of time. What if something was needed (an emergency)? Susan would be trapped and so would Matthew.

I started to do some work and get back to the real world of making the business go, trying to find customers and come up with a plan to protect us (the staff) from whatever will happen at the health care system where I am employed.

I tried to reach her rehab physician to "pin her down" about the phrase, "I'm still optimistic." What does that mean? Have they written Susan off (walking as a goal)? Just a basic fundamental question. Susan needs a straightforward answer.

I was in a meeting when my secretary called to tell me Susan's doctor was on the line. While I followed along with what was being said during our phone conversation, there are still some unanswered issues for me. Regardless, this is the gist of the conversation:

> *"Susan has no idea where her left leg is or what she does with it during exercises. Therefore, she, in effect, has no use of it because there is no sensation of 'where it is.' She is sensitive to touch, but not to movement or position. Thus, how can she ever walk?"*

> *"She has good muscle tone in her leg. That's necessary for walking to be a possibility. Usually sensation precedes tone. Didn't happen in this case.*

> *"Her arm has improved vis-à-vis sensation. Initially, she did not know where it was, but now she does. A real marked improvement over when she first arrived. They have not seen such improvement in the leg, but expect to see some. When, how much, and how quickly is anybody's guess.*

> *"Therefore, there is hope—we just have to hope that it does come back."*

> *Nothing is for sure but hope – without hope there is nothing; one might as well hope.*

December 11 - Friday: 10:45 p.m.

My Mother is still sore (legs and body). Too much lifting, walking, tension, and lack of sleep. The past month has just beaten her up. I was off yesterday and took off today to give my mom a break. I have the time coming from work, so I might as well use it.

What's happened since Wednesday? For one thing, there was a 7" snow storm Wednesday and Wednesday night. Sort of funny that all along I predicted a "snow storm" on Matthew's

94

original due date, December 10th, and that is what happened! I'm better than the meteorologist at long-range forecasting.

I talked with Susan Wednesday night and she sounded upbeat. She has an amazing attitude to keep going, in spite of her limitations and the recent gloomy news regarding the ability to walk. We have to be positive and hopeful—there is no other choice. Also, there is some optimism given what Dr. Smith discussed with us. That's what keeps us going. Any small slice of hope is better than doom and gloom. Everything will turn out ok. We might as well be positive while we wait.

I stayed home Thursday. Dora was off and I wanted to help my mother with Matthew. I did some grocery shopping and running around. I also cleaned the house. Alisa came over and stayed with Matthew while mother and I went shopping to Field's.

We still need to Christmas shop—so life goes on—we have to keep everything going while we wait for Susan to come home. I was able to leave home and get downtown early Thursday afternoon. I went to Susan's speech class.

The rehab staff is trying to figure out what cognitive challenges, if any, Susan has. She tried to solve a math problem. Math wasn't her favorite subject in school. Although she earned an A in college algebra. She had an extremely difficult time trying to figure out what to do let alone the answer.

The question: "If you were going to drive to Dallas and it was 500 miles away and you were going to drive 50 miles per hour – how many hours would it take you to drive to Dallas?"

I was sitting off to the side and could see Susan "thinking through" the elements of the question. She had taken the law school entrance exam and passed it by answering far more difficult questions, but this was a life test with a lot more riding on it.

Times had changed and this question needed an answer – she asked to have the question repeated – bought time but little else.

Finally, after what seemed an eternity the speech therapist asked, "Susan, do you know the answer? How many hours?"

Susan sat still – emotionless – finally a slight smile crossed her lips as she said, "No I don't know how many hours it would take. Besides I'd fly and would not waste my time driving – let alone driving to Dallas of all places. Just like the Millionaire Quiz Show – this is my final answer."

Susan turned to me and said, "I'm done – let's go."

Though the session had just started and was to last for an hour it abruptly ended. She was done and I wheeled her out of the office back into the hallway. The therapist never said a word.

Later we talked. She had felt extreme pressure to perform because I was present and then felt embarrassed because she couldn't answer the word problem. Somehow she is "stupid" now, therefore, I must be embarrassed because she is "dumb." That's how she sees it, but that's not the case. She's not dumb! As I told her "I wouldn't go to Dallas either."

We talked about what had happened. There is nothing to be embarrassed about. This is easy for me to say, hard for her to accept. Each task she is asked to do that is difficult or impossible for her to do robs her of self-esteem. I told her that if I did or said things that made her feel diminished in someway, she needed to let me know. Or, if she wanted to do things herself, that was fine with me. I wanted her to understand that I respected her autonomy and independence and would provide help, if needed and/or requested. Susan runs her life. No one else does or should even try.

Susan talked about how difficult it was having me help her dress to go out for the walk we took Thursday night to get some fresh air. She is almost totally dependent on me, the exact opposite of the take-charge person she was, and as I reminded her, will become again. I understand her point; it's a delicate balance to strike; the compromise between needing help and feeling helpless; asking for assistance and someone taking over your life. The issue of asking for help is also a difficult task. These are issues that will always be with us and ones that we both have to be sensitive about. For now the rule is: she will ask if she needs help. I will help if asked, and I will try to stop hovering waiting to be asked. My intentions, while laudable, clash with my behavior. I need to back off until called upon. Susan wonders how trainable I am.

We also discussed the issue of full-time help for her and Matthew. Once she is home, somebody is going to have to take care of them when I am not home or when I travel. There is no way around the need to have full-time help. For example, I just can't run out to the store with her home alone with Matthew. What could she do if there was an emergency? What could she do period—if Matthew was in trouble—or there was a fire—or who knows what? Knowing this intellectually and coming to accept it are vastly different places in one's sense of self. This issue of help, like many other issues, will take time to sort through and in all probability will never be fully resolved. This is a life-long process of learning to redefine our lives.

This is a reality we have to confront and formulate a "strategy" that is workable for all parties. This is especially true when I travel, which I'll have to do. Someone will have to stay overnight.

We had a nice visit last night. Time always seems to fly when we are together. We reviewed both of our days—what's coming up and the plans for the weekend. She can come home both Saturday and Sunday which is great for us and great for her and Matthew. They can get re-acquainted and Susan can get acclimated to home. She will have to go back at night. She likes to characterize her visit as a "work release program" – she can have home visits but can't stay. So up and back we will go for this weekend pass, staying as long as possible without being classified as AWOL.

Susan will have her hair styled tomorrow at the salon. That should make her feel good. Joyce is going to take the baby overnight. That will be a trick, to pack up for an overnighter; clothes, bottles, diapers, etc., to travel, along with the bassinet.

Matthew is up to drinking 3.5 ounces. That amount really knocks him out. He is sleeping well with a full stomach and growing each day.

Susan called this morning. She was able to bend her left leg back towards her chest for the first time. This is a significant step forward. She is still waiting for sensation to return, and then she can move forward with walking. But gross motor movement is the first step before fine motor control.

December 13 - Sunday: 4:30 p.m.

Susan has been home both Saturday and today. She cannot have an overnight pass until Christmas Eve. But at least she can get out each weekend.

Matthew stayed overnight with Joyce and Chris; that's a big help because I can sleep and try and get some things done before I head downtown to pick up Susan.

My mother has been with Betty for the weekend. That will give her a good break from the workload and responsibilities.

Susan mentioned how, at times, she gets terrified at the thought of not walking, standing or ever using her left arm. "When these thoughts occur, I get physically sick. It doesn't happen often, but when it does, it is overwhelming."

There is great joy for Susan in getting home, sitting and doing nothing. It's a relief to be out—home looks great! Even when there are things to do and you'd like to fix up the house, the home looks like a castle when you've been away so long.

I brought her home and got things going, like checking out the baby's room and the mail, the wash and things like that. Since Matthew was with Joyce, we went there for a few hours until Susan's hair appointment.

It is difficult for Susan to accept other people caring for Matthew when she can't. The loss is magnified when you see others enjoying him, caring for him while you're on the sidelines. It is hard to convey the pain I see in her face – glad to see him happy – sad because she is not the one making him happy – not yet. But that time will come. It has to.

A simple thing like hugging can't be done the way she use to do it. No more two arm hugs! But to have her one arm around me is comforting.

December 14 - Monday: 7:30 p.m.

I stayed home in the morning because Mother needed a good night's rest. She stayed by my sister, Betty. Dora came early (8:30 a.m.). I made a few calls from home before I got organized and started the day.

I finally got to work at 9:30 a.m. There were many things to catch up with, such as memos and phone calls. I also worked on the insurance claim forms which is quite a project given all the paperwork that has to be filed and re-filed before payment is made for anything.

I began preparing documents for Social Security, worker's disability and private insurance applications. Someone once said that insurance is 95% process and 5% substance, meaning that there is little needed information, it just takes countless numbers of forms and hours to obtain payment for a claim. I certainly understand that now.

I completed the paperwork to obtain Susan's medical record. She has a six-week OB/Gyn check-up soon. The doctor Susan selected said she had tried to locate her records, but couldn't. They were out (not available). Makes me wonder where and who has the records! Why are they "out" and unavailable?

I talked with an attorney who suggested that he would "oversee" the case if we choose his firm to investigate this matter. Since retainers are not typical, a percentage of the settlement is the way fees are determined. This lawyer suggested we needed a firm to oversee the lawyers. What a crazy world, "who can you trust?" I am supposed to hire a law firm to make sure the law firm I hire for the case has our interests as the primary concern. Maybe I should hire someone to oversee the overseer.

I am having a difficult time coming to terms with what has happened. I was walking around the grocery store tonight in a trance. No matter how many things got done today, there is still more to do. Will we ever get back to the way it was? I know the answer, but prefer to believe it is possible.

I talked with Susan. She sounded like she had a good day. The PT/OT people from the Rehab Institute are planning to come out Wednesday at noon to check out the home and see what we need and/or should get done to accommodate the disability. Still evaluating what type of wheelchair may or may not work. Susan will be coming home with the rehab staff to participate in a review of what is possible to make the house more accessible.

I talked with the Social Security Administration about the disability application. There are mounds of paperwork, more forms, more documents, and more time to spend in this seemingly unending sea of questions and documents. The process of applying is extremely difficult. I know that even if there is a minor mistake made during completion of these forms someone will find it, flag it, reject the application and we will be told to start anew.

Susan went from her psychotherapy session into the PT/exercise class. She took her first step today; locked her left leg, shifted her weight to her right leg and then brought the left leg along. "One small step," she said. Hope continues! She was ecstatic. Having accomplished the impossible – she worried about whether or not she could repeat the feat.

Even though I had a two-day break from Matthew, I am exhausted. I think it's all the running around, all the pressure to do everything that nobody else will or can or I won't let do. It's the "on call" state that is tiring. Everybody needs some help sooner or later and I am in the later camp for the time being. Everybody wants to help us but it is even more work to coordinate the "help." I am now known as "Mr. No." Every time someone offers to help I say "No – that's ok, I can do it."

Mother is getting even more tired. She started to talk about the next stage—who will take over when Susan gets home? If I had that answer, I'd be a genius. I don't have a clue. As my mother said, "I never thought it would be more than two weeks." If only it was over in two weeks. Who knew anything about what would happen? Will happen? There was no prior experience with a stroke and the rehab necessary to regain functioning by which to judge time and progress. Things will take time and no one knows any more than that. "I thought it would be over," my Mother stated. In two weeks no less; it is not over—it is just starting!

Another night is ahead. Soon I will be asleep. However, I awake to the reality that Susan is not home – she is not the Susan she was, but she still is the Susan I love. So I stop thinking about things because it just takes time, time away from things that could be done and need to be done—just do what needs to be done. What we had is gone – it's gone forever – I need to focus my energy on what can/might be. Thinking about the past, what we did, what our plans were is not helpful. It is a waste of time. "The past is only useful if it helps you go forward." That is my motto. Forward is where we are going. What lies ahead is far more important than where we were or have been. We cannot predict the future, we can't change the past. I remember a quote Susan told me years ago that I often use in classes I teach: "Some people prefer the certainty of misery to the mercy of uncertainty." I need to stay in the present and I will do all right.

December 16 - Wednesday: 11:40 a.m.

Susan is coming home for a visit with two of her therapists to check out the house for her wheelchair and other adaptive equipment like grab bars in the bath area. At least she can go for a ride and get out of the hospital. Also, these therapists will offer parenting suggestions/child care tips. Since they are single and do not have children it will be interesting to listen to their suggestions.

I talked to a lawyer today about reviewing what had transpired during the delivery. The firm seems interested and suggested a time for us to visit. I think it is best Susan and I go to them, rather than have them come to the rehab center and stir up controversy. An interesting thing happened as we talked. When the lawyer asked the doctor's name, I said "Randell," and she filled in the last name without me saying it. "We have had a number of judgments against him," she said. Needless to say, I was shocked, and Susan will be stunned!

I went to work yesterday. Quite busy lining up business and working on various grants. The day goes by quickly, but with little sleep at night and returning home to start all over again, it is a grueling schedule.

Susan has reached her limit with the hospital stay—the institutionalization aspect of it is getting to her. At times, she is so overwhelmed by the nature of the hospitalization that she does not know if she can tolerate it any longer. Also, she really hasn't regained much use of her left leg or arm. In fact, the other day, as she grabbed her arm she realized it was the arm of the nursing attendant. It is this type of "reality shock" that destroy her hopes. Hard to be positive when these types of things happen.

The ladies from rehab (OT and PT) brought Susan home to check out the house and what she can or cannot do. It's amazing how naïve and out of touch with reality these women are. Both are single young women with no parenting experience. There are certain things Susan can do, and other things she can't. To make it appear she is able to "do it all" is a painful charade— everyone knows she can't, but we pretend otherwise. Susan is the only one who knows the reality of the situation and prefers to confront it rather than to pretend otherwise.

The occupational therapist felt Susan could change Matthew's diaper with one hand. All that needs to happen is: 1) Susan would lift him out of the crib after putting the rail down; 2) he would have to lay still of course – fat chance this would happen; 3) she would open the new diaper and ask him to position himself on it so it can be closed – might as well have him change it for himself. I forgot, should the diaper have a surprise? That was not covered.

Fortunately, the home occupational and physical therapists are mothers who can offer practical advice and suggest strategies that might be helpful in Susan's role as a mother. Also, the home therapists know what it is like to be a mother and can be a sounding board for Susan. She has to talk to someone about these issues and these therapists seem willing to talk.

December 20 - Sunday: 11:50 a.m.

It's Sunday. Susan is on a home pass like yesterday. The baby is at Pat's (a sister-in-law). Today, we will put up the Christmas tree. Her mom and dad, plus the girls are coming over. So, we'll have dinner and enjoy the day. The eternal optimist!

Given all that has been going on things are going well. Every step Susan takes is impressive, especially since the initial judgment was she would not walk. A major victory for Susan! She is able to do a few additional things (more range of motion exercises with her arm and leg) and this is remarkable progress. Our hope is that further gains can be made. We hope more functioning and use of her hand and leg will return over time. The key point to note is that these increasing small steps improve one's sense of self- worth, as well as demonstrate progress.

That is not to say that things couldn't be better. Susan feels the frustration of being dependent for nearly everything, and rightly so. The personal struggle of old self versus the to-be-defined evolving self continues. In this constant comparative mindset Susan always is behind where she currently is. It would be impossible to be otherwise. Nevertheless, believing that you are falling short of the mark all the time is taxing. Setting the bar high is Susan's style.

Time is still scarce—that's an understatement. Activities should calm down when Susan returns home, but there is still the responsibility to orchestrate everything and to think about all that has to be done, taken with, and packed up or whatever. I try not to let myself think about what new demands will be made on "time" when we are a family at home again. To be a family again is the goal, the demands and tasks will fall into place.

I watched a "recovery-focused" show on TV about rehab patients. It presented a wide variety of cases with varying disabilities. Each in their own way demonstrated spirit and determination and unbelievable courage – attributes that Susan possesses.

A few ideas and perspectives were interesting on the show. The point repeatedly made throughout was that "a bad moment or bad day does not mean it is a bad life." An interesting perspective, I plan to remember this point of view because I am sure it will be helpful to recall. Susan already has embraced this philosophy.

Otto and Viola had arrived early in the day. We had to get the tree up, find the lights and ornaments and get it all together.

While I started with the Christmas tree, Matthew returned from his overnight stay with Pat and Bill, Susan's aunt and her husband, who seemed to have enjoyed caring for him. It's a help to have people pitch in like they have done.

The girls came by and we all had dinner. I'm getting good at cooking and all the rest. Dinner must have been good, because there was so little left.

After a few hours, things quieted down and there was silence in the home. Great sound, to hear nothing. Susan, Matthew, and I napped.

Mother and Betty came by about 6:00 p.m. They watched Matthew while I took Susan back to rehab.

Susan's about had it. I know I have mentioned this matter before. But every day, the level of frustration, loneliness, and profound sadness of being away from home becomes increasingly difficult to bear. She is fed up with rehab; enough is enough! She is depressed about not being able to care for Matthew. Not being able to be with Matthew. Immediately after her brain surgery, Susan wanted to be able to breast feed Matthew. She knew how important this was and was determined to try. But she was unable to do so. She cried for hours. Life is moving on and she doesn't feel she is. She doesn't feel she is aboard the train. Life left her at the hospital and she has been trying to catch up. She will. I have no doubt she will, but the long view is hard to accept when you are in the moment – the here and now. This is also easy for me to say, much harder for her to believe, at least at this point in time.

There is no way she can make up for the loss of the seven weeks that have passed since the stroke. She has expressed that sentiment more than once. "Matthew doesn't even know me. How could he since I am not there for him. He sees strangers more than me." Her hopes and plans can't be fulfilled—not in her present condition. It is just impossible for her (at this time), given her arm and leg, to do anything but try and get stronger. That task is daunting enough. Saying that and accepting it (moving on) are very different and difficult tasks.

In some ways, I think, Susan could accept her limitations if she could take care of Matthew. Not being able to do so is the cruelest twist to this daily nightmare. Every time she realizes what she herself can't do, it only magnifies the level of her disappointment. If the basics of feeding and changing can't be done now, how can the chasing, playing, and exploring be accomplished? Easy to say "don't think of it, in time you'll be back to your old self," etc. None of those empty platitudes help when confronted with the reality of limitations. However, belief in getting better and adapting to the disability provides hope that will sustain her.

What has been missed or lost by Susan pales in comparison to all that will be lost, or at least changed, in the future. It is a personal, deeply felt loss that I can only imagine. The goal is to enjoy the moment, enjoy it for what it is and for what she is able to do. The past and the future are out of our control, thus experience the moment - that is what truly counts. Focus on the present. That is all any of us really has.

December 21 - Monday: 6:00 a.m.

Matthew settled down about 11:30 p.m. last night and got up about 4:00 a.m. He was real congested and one eye was closed with a crusty discharge. Nose drops helped clear his congestion. A warm, wet cloth loosened the crusted material from his eye so he could open it. I held him for awhile after this morning feeding and then he went down. I talk to him about Susan. He has an intense look on his face as I speak. I'm sure it's my voice, but I also like to believe that he is keenly interested in Mom and desperately wants to know how things are going. So he and I have a "daily update" on how Mom is doing.

Since it was 5:00 a.m. when Matthew went back to sleep, I stayed up. I paid bills, took Hans for a walk, and did the wash. I might as well be productive when I can. Can't wait to see how alert I'll be during the rest of the day.

Susan called at 1:14 p.m. and left a message. "I took sixteen steps today—not too bad, huh! Talk to you later." Best message I had heard in a long time.

I called Susan back a few minutes after her call. "Sixteen? Only sixteen" I said. "Maybe it was 17, not sure because I took so many steps," Susan responded. This is our unique way of giving support and congratulations in a backhanded way. She was elated and so was I. This is what we had hoped for. A small step is not small when you couldn't do it before.

On the other hand, the excitement is bittersweet. This is not walking like we know walking to be. It is not what we had or what we want. In an ironic way, we're excited about what we hope will change quickly. But the real source of the excitement is the symbol of success and courage this and these steps represent. The work, effort and determination cannot be measured in steps. It's not quitting and still trying that says more than steps can. It's the determination and a resolve to be who she was that speaks volumes about who Susan is. These are qualities she has always had. They are just being applied to issues and tasks that we never thought we would experience.

December 23 - Wednesday: 8:30 p.m.

I just finished cleaning the house for Christmas Eve. I will do the floors and vacuum tomorrow. Hope all goes well with seventeen people in our home.

Yesterday (Tuesday, December 22), I went downtown to spend the day with Susan. I attended her classes and saw the routine she goes through each day. I saw her walk (25 steps). She was afraid she couldn't do it again, or do it in front of me. But she was successful. The smile on her face was all you needed to see to know how much this meant to her. Her smile lit up the room.

Determination is an understated word to describe the effort Susan puts forth in standing and walking. She has had to relearn every phase of this task from standing, muscle tightening, to foot placement, etc., and mentally repeat these elements of walking every time she takes a step. Nothing is automatic or natural; everything must be done in sequence and done over and over again with each step. It is thinking through what was taken for granted each time she takes a step that makes walking possible. All this is occurring in spite of the fact that she cannot feel or locate her left leg. Taking a step is an act of faith. If she does all the mental stages in sequence, the foot will be where it has to be in order for her to take a step. Just as quickly she has to be prepared to do it again and again.

Took 25 steps today! It's like a marathon—she is exhausted after such an effort.

I spent time in her classes. We had lunch and then Susan asked to visit Olsen and Passavant, where she had been prior to rehab. She wanted to see where she had been and what the place and people were like. Susan doesn't remember all that happened or who was involved in her care. So it was a chance to retrace steps. It is also a chance to see places, rooms, and hallways that will be discussed over and over. To see people who cared for her. To have an opportunity to thank them.

It was emotional for both of us. It was difficult for me to see those places and remember the feelings and pain that were associated with them. It was a good thing for her to do—sort of fill in the blanks over the past seven weeks.

We started at Olsen where I first found her on the Neuro Intensive Care Unit. We saw Rick and Steve who had both taken care of her during her stay. Susan remembered Steve. They both expressed how nice it was to see someone healthy, given who they work with on a daily bases. They were grateful that Susan took the time to visit the unit. As she said, "I have so many things and people to be grateful for. I just had to come by."

We stopped at Passavant on the fourth floor to visit the two nursing stations where she spent time after her surgery. Susan remembered some of this experience; she was not sure of Room 458. We saw a few of the nurses: Kimberly, Kelly, and Ruby. All were real pleased to see Susan.

On the way back, we stopped at the high-risk nursery to see some of the nurses who cared for Matthew: Kathy, Gina, Tina and the social worker, Colleen. All were happy to see us. It's clear that with many patients the nurses are left wondering what happened. It's nice to be able to personally thank them for their help and the care they gave Matthew.

We returned to rehab in time for the 1:30 OT class. They "bowled" and played the "hangman game." Seems like an awfully sick game to play on a rehab unit. When you look around and see the extent of the impairments these individuals have, you can only imagine what it must do to them and their families to see them engaged in "bowling with a balloon." But you can only do what you can do—which is more than could be done a few days ago. So progress and the direction of progress is moving forward. That is the key direction – forward.

We spent time in the exercise class with Richard. Paula, her PT, arranged a fitting for a walking brace. The brace will help keep Susan's left leg straight now that she has a sense of where the leg is and can move it. The brace will both support the leg and knee and keep it from flopping around. The brace will also support her ankle and foot. Susan can take a few steps without the brace, but it is best to wear it all the time.

Today, we had the 4:00 p.m. appointment with the lawyers. We took a cab there and back. We spent about 1½ hours with them, reviewing the events surrounding Susan's disability. Our guess is they (the firm) will take the case.

The cab ride was interesting. The pickup at rehab was okay; there was no curb so Susan could easily enter the car. But the return trip was challenging. The cab stopped by a curb. Susan could not get in as easily because she can't go down curbs. There was no room between the cab and the curb. Susan could not take a step down (off the curb) and then into the cab. Somehow she got positioned so she could just fall into the cab (as I lowered her into the back seat) and we were on our way back. Almost broke her leg and ankle, but thankfully, that didn't happen. The ride in the cab heightened my awareness of barriers to walking – getting around that I would never have noticed in a million years. Now the radar is on.

December 29 - Tuesday: 1:05 p.m. (at work)

Guess why I didn't write for the past few days? Time—absolutely right—no time. I know it's trite to keep saying that, but this "no time" is an overwhelming feeling to contend with since I'm always running late or have more things to do than there is time to do them. The faster one runs the further behind one gets. I need to figure out what can get done and forget the rest – if only for the moment.

Let's try and catch up on the ever-changing landscape of events. First, the best news is that Susan is coming home December 31, 1992, instead of January 5, 1993. The overnight Christmas visit convinced her that she had to get home. Institutional life and being institutionalized is just more than she can handle—enough is enough. I am sure Susan said she would be leaving one way or the other, with or without the hospital's blessing. Regardless, the discharge – home-coming date is set.

Dr. Smith agreed and she is preparing for Susan's discharge. With the upcoming end-of-the-year celebration and weekend, it is not that easy to be discharged and get started with a full home care program. Susan will probably miss a few days. Nothing will be occurring at rehab over the holiday so it makes sense to sit at home rather than in the hospital.

Christmas Eve worked out well. Susan's mother worked very hard to organize and prepare all the special foods. As always, there was far too much food and 17 people filled the house, especially with our space, the wheelchair and Matthew's stuff.

All-in-all everything went smoothly, but I was exhausted from trying to clean, organize the house, get Susan, help with the food and gifts, get drinks, feed Matthew, etc. There are not enough hands and bodies to get everything done.

People came about 4:30 p.m. and left around 11:30 p.m. I always have this fear over how such an event will turn out – is it just too much to do? But it all seems to work out in the end. Joyce, Carole and my sisters helped clean up and take care of Matthew.

Gifts! To say there was a mountain of gifts is to seriously understate the true number of presents. Everyone was very generous with us and Matthew. The clothes and toys make it impossible to move in the house. Matthew already has more than he needs or can reasonably use and he is only seven weeks old.

Melinda gave Susan an incredible ring: Matthew's birthstone with three diamonds surrounding it for the three of us. She always comes up with these unique and thoughtful gifts. Also, she bought an array of outfits for Matthew. He'll never be able to wear all these clothes, since they are the same size and there are only so many times in a day you can change him.

I helped Susan get ready for bed by 11:45 p.m.

(I just got a call from home. Dora and
Mother fell down some stairs in the basement, trying

to get the buggy up. I'm going to the house and will continue the story later.)

December 30 - Wednesday: 6:40 p.m.

Somehow nobody got hurt—a miracle. Dora has a black and blue butt. My mother has a scratch on her hand and that's it. I called her last night and this morning. She's fine. Dora is fine. Have I ever said, never a dull moment?

Back to Christmas Eve. Matthew had been up all evening, so he was exhausted. Seems funny to say that I helped Susan get ready for bed, but that is the case. Not sure how her being dependent on me will affect our relationship. Hope it doesn't. But it just feels unnatural to have to take care of her. I don't like the feeling or the responsibility—hopefully, it's temporary. You can imagine how she feels. I am not sure what to do, what help she would like (if any), or how to even bring up the topic. Trial and error will have to be the guide.

Getting into bed is not what it was. She needs help. Pillows to support her arm and a hand brace has to be secured around her waist so her shoulder and arm will roll with her as she rolls. Nevertheless, we got through all those things and lay next to each other. It had been a long time—it seemed like forever.

What used to be spontaneous is now planned, discussed, and positioned; but making love, the feelings, the desires are there. Those will never change.

Matthew got up at 6:00 a.m. on Christmas Day. I fed him and he and I went back to bed. Susan and I got up about 8:00 a.m. Matthew had received cards from his parents. His first Christmas cards. We opened and read them like we had never seen them before. We just sat enjoying the moment and the home.

We called Harry (he used to be a patient at rehab) and he was glad to hear from us. It sounds like he is doing okay at the retirement center. He had to leave his apartment because he couldn't take care of himself. A very kind man, in his late 60s, will never be able to live independently again.

By 9:30-10:00 a.m., we decided to start getting ready, so we could be at my sister's by 1:30 p.m. In short, we didn't make it.

As Susan said, at least two of the three of us were clean (she and Matthew). I came back home to clean up. It is hard to comprehend all that has to be done to be responsible for two people. Bathing, dressing and washing; getting coats on and carrying everything to the car. It is challenging. Total care is on me and it's oppressing at times because there is so much to do and think about that I become immobilized. I have to realize that what I can do is good enough. To do more is impossible. To expect to do more is unrealistic. I need to think about going easier than I have. The feeling of being behind doesn't make things go easier or faster.

Susan took two hours from start to finish, Matthew used one hour, and it took 45 minutes to gather up all that had to be brought over to my sister's and load it into the car. In between care-giving, I'm cleaning the floor, doing dishes, picking up, washing clothes and laying out clothes to wear, etc.

I was exhausted. Then I returned home and got ready myself, after taking the dog for a walk and giving him his food and water. My sister called to see where I was, as if I fell asleep. Guess they thought I could be a little quicker than I was.

Betty had a great meal. She always goes all out, plus there were all the presents; the second round of presents. By 7:30 p.m., we had to start back. Matthew stayed overnight because I was going to drive Susan back to rehab.

Leaving Matthew and returning to rehab are heavy burdens. In the car, she decided that she couldn't stay until January 5. There would be no real therapy for New Year's Eve or Day, plus the Saturday and Sunday, which followed those days. All she would be doing is going back and forth. All that would occur is her sleeping at rehab—nothing else.

Saturday we visited her brother and Matthew stayed overnight. Friday night I had back pain which made it difficult to stand. I took two Advil and gratefully, it went away. I lay in bed saying I can't get sick. Thinking I had a disc problem led to a massive headache, and fortunately both went away. If they hadn't, I don't know what I'd have done.

Susan was even stronger about her desire to leave rehab, as we returned last Sunday to the hospital (12/27/92). I can't really blame her. Her argument is excellent, sound, and as it turned out, would be accepted by Dr. Smith.

Melinda came by rehab on Sunday for a visit. I prepared sandwiches for them. Melinda replaced the charm with Matthew's picture that was accidentally discarded early in the hospitalization. During a changing of the gown, someone failed to take it off and it was lost in the hospital wash. Melinda always comes up with very thoughtful gifts. So she replaced the charm necklace.

On the Sunday after Christmas as we were leaving home to return to rehab, Susan indicated she was leaving rehab. Enough was enough. In her mind she was done – was getting out. "I can't do this anymore. It is as simple as that."

I went to work Monday and got the call at 8:20 a.m. She was being discharged on December 31, 1992. I stopped at the "Y" to clear out my locker. It was a sad moment. I miss not exercising, playing racquetball and just working out. That's gone for awhile, until we figure out ways of doing it.

I took care of insurance calls and paperwork while at work. It is hard to really get any work done. Add the holidays to the mix and even less work is doable. There is no time to focus on projects (let alone unpack from an internal office move) with everything that is occurring. I try to fit some work in whenever I can.

I took Matthew, Mother, and Alisa out to dinner on Tuesday and to Marshall Field's. This was sort of an outing. Hard to believe all the stuff you have to haul along for fun: buggy, bag, food, change of clothes, etc. I fed Matthew while Alisa and mother shopped. He was wide-eyed about all the sights and sounds he was seeing for the first time.

Matthew spit up quite a bit. There was too much bouncing around. It is hard to change his clothes and diaper during the outing, plus repack everything (him, the bags, and the buggy) into the car. I'm sure, with time, all this activity will become second nature (I hope so).

I was gone about 3-3½ hours and it felt like 25. The tension and responsibility to organize, think of, and pull off these outings is there. As I say, in time, they'll become second nature.

Today I was up at 5:15 a.m. and stayed up. Hans had to go out. Mother and Matthew got up at 6:15 a.m. I fed him and he fell back asleep while Mother and I cleaned up and packed up. She is finished with her "tour of duty." The entire car was loaded with food, gifts, clothes, luggage, coats, and boots. Mother had been here since November 14th —almost seven weeks. It was time to go home.

I worry about her. This experience and the work have aged her. She really has suffered due to the tension of caring for Matthew, just not being in a comfortable environment and her old routine. I hope over time, she can regain her old self. This is the first time I ever heard her say she felt her age.

I got everything together and left the house at 9:17 a.m. to shop, take her home, and head back for lunch with Rossi, a research colleague of mine. Matthew will have to be a traveler. He has no choice, because where I need to go, he'll go.

Matthew did well today. My mother gave him a bath before the trip back home. We really have to just get organized and get going. I didn't want to have the girls or anyone watch him. He just has to learn to go with the flow—and he does real well.

Susan called my mother to thank her for all her help, all she had done for us and, especially, Matthew. "I'm not sure how to put into words my thanks and appreciation for what you have done," Susan said. Later Susan told me that: "I just tried to thank her, but we were both crying so much it was hard to tell if either side understood what the other was trying to say."

My Mother is clearly happy to be home, but equally sad over leaving Matthew. She won't see him or play with him every day like she had been doing. She'll miss that, in spite of all the tension and work that was involved in caring for him.

I called to tell her Matthew was a good boy at lunch. I knew she'd wonder and want to know. Dora called and checked up on how things were going.

It's the night before the last day at rehab—no more sleeping at rehab after tonight.

Anxious, excited, scared, confident, unsure of the future, sort of a mixed bag of feelings and emotions. I'm accustomed to seeing and remembering Susan as she was. It is very difficult to see her in so much emotional turmoil. I'm sure these feelings are magnified for her.

The home is a reminder of what was and what needs to be done. Real mix of emotions: joy being back, but not back in any way that you wanted to be or had hoped to be. But back she is and here is where we will start our life's journey. Perhaps continue is a better word. We have already started the journey, just had a slight detour.

Chapter 6
HOME? THIS IS HOME

"We deem those happy who from the experience of life have learned to bear its ills, without being overcome by them.

- Juvenal

January 1, 1993 - Friday: 10:30 a.m.

Susan was discharged New Year's Eve, so the year ended great and we have high hopes for 1993. Given the progress she has made in two weeks (from not walking at all to walking 80 feet), we are very optimistic.

Susan became upset with me as we were leaving rehab; she felt that I was "on edge and ready to blow," which makes her feel uncomfortable. She feels that I am, in effect, fed up with her. Since she is unable to do a lot, this "edge" I have makes for a tense and anxious situation. I am not upset, I am over my head and lack patience – a bad combination. I hope to be known as "easy-going" Bill soon.

We talked about what to do to make the situation less tense. I told her I hate helping, because it reminds me of what she has lost. Not hating her, but the fact she has to go through such a struggle. My anger really doesn't come out very well. There is an insight for you!

A key thing for me to come to grips with is just how much I can do and when I have to take a time-out. I do not see Susan as dependent on me, but rather as needing some help. This makes us peers versus I/she feeling like I have to take charge of her life. That is the last thing I need to do or she wants.

The way little things are done makes all the difference. Like her coat. She needs help with her arm and to get it on right, but I don't have to put her hood up, she can decide if she is cold and wants her hood up. That's the difference between helping and deciding. I can tell you that it's a fine line—but one that you have to work out to keep the relationship and balance going.

Obviously, we have to talk about these and many other issues all the time. I have to be easier with just taking my time and not getting on Hans or Matthew. I know there are times when I feel like one more thing is too much. It's impossible to do everything—I have to stand back and let it go—not become overwhelmed—maybe easier said than done. But in taking a moment to reflect before speaking, it is surprising how much easier it is to get things done. It is certainly a joke to consider myself

116

overwhelmed. Susan in her sarcastic way pointedly asks, "You're overwhelmed?" That comment is a great reality check for me!

Saying goodbye to Dr. Smith and the staff who helped her at RIC was very hard for Susan. These people, especially Paula, have given Susan her life back. The chance/opportunity to walk and regain her functioning. What greater gift can there be—a chance.

Chris and Joyce (Susan's brother and his wife) and Della and Bob (friends) came by for a drink before going out to dinner on New Year's Eve. Nice to visit with them. Dressed Matthew in his tux outfit and took some pictures. Hope they turn out.

All-in-all, a good end to the old year and a great start to the New Year. What lies before us is uncertain ,but what is certain is that we will find it together. Susan is home. We are a family. Onward we go.

January 6 - Wednesday: 8:50 p.m.

I'm in the waiting area of the ICU – ER unit at Lutheran General Hospital. Susan had multiple seizures starting at 6:00 p.m., Monday, January 4. These were generalized seizures where the whole body becomes extremely rigid and the person loses contact with their surroundings.

That evening we started to eat dinner at about 5:30 p.m. with her mom and dad. At 5:45, Susan said she wasn't feeling well. As I looked at her, her eyes were shallow, like she was not really seeing me; there was a twitch to her face; and, a tremor to her hand. Even I knew things didn't look good.

I tried to reassure her while I found the number to rehab and, unbelievably, got through to Renee, her nurse at rehab, and to Dr. Smith. We talked about what was happening. Susan talked to Dr. Smith, and it was clear to me that we had to go to the hospital. Whatever was going on didn't look like it was "normal." This was not going to pass. It was a seizure. I have never seen one before. For the brain to be under attack and out of control is terrifying. The seizure seizes your life at that moment. There is no choice; no will power can stop the seizure. The seizure will do what is pleases for how long it wishes.

I found out later that about 5:00 p.m. (a half hour before we started the dinner) Susan had felt lightheaded and experienced the room spinning. Anyway, things were going downhill and we had to get on our way to the hospital.

While I felt there were 1,000 things to do all at the same time, I realized I had to get her dressed (get her coat on while she is rigid), get her into the car (when she can't stand or walk), and get on the way to the hospital. Her parents would watch Matthew. They would call my sister to come and stay with him. I found her medical discharge summary and her coat, wheelchair, wallet, keys, etc. She was rigid and had a hard time standing or walking. So I carried her into the garage and carefully put her in the front seat of the car.

She was nauseated, so I took a bowl along. Of course, it was snowing and messy outside along with the rush-hour traffic. She wasn't easy to move around; more like dead weight. Susan was unable to support her weight. Susan wasn't tracking like she had been doing—not aware of her surroundings, non-responsive to questions, etc..

As we drove, I tried to engage her in conversation; tried to figure out if she was "here" or out "there"—halfway to the hospital, she had multiple generalized seizures in the car while I was driving.

The terror and fear I felt was palpable. What should I do? Stop at the fire department or police station that I passed on the way to the hospital, or would that waste more time than if I kept driving on to the hospital? She started to roll her eyes, became so rigid like she was stretching while sitting, drool was on the side of her mouth. I grabbed her by the jacket so she wouldn't slide down in the seat and be choked by the seat belt. I put my arm across her chest and grabbed the seat belt strap to "hold her in place," while continuing to drive on.

A lifetime seemed to go by and I thought she was going to die, it (the seizure) lasted about 20-30 seconds. She came out of it and could talk and knew who I was—what a relief! I was never so glad to hear her say my name than at that moment.

Susan experienced multiple seizures on the way to the ER. Upon arrival and hearing the history the doctor on call was concerned that a re-bleed had occurred. I couldn't believe it, that another bleed could possibly occur. The CAT scan showed no new problems, thank God. Why were these seizures happening? "We don't know" was the ER physician's answer. "However, the scan did reveal a mass – perhaps related to the recent surgery where the residual blood is not re-absorbed." Now that is something to consider, a cloudy mass. The word "mass" I translate to tumor. A new issue I thought – a brain tumor.

Joyce and Chris came to the ER (glad they were there) to see Susan. While talking with them, Susan rolled her eyes, stared at the wall, began to drool, and had to have saliva vacuumed from her mouth. It was very hard to see her so out of it—so very afraid. I can't imagine how she felt as her mind – mental abilities were assaulted by these relentless seizures. She knows something is not right in her head, but is powerless to do anything about it.

Susan was admitted and was moved to ICU about 11:00 p.m. I stayed for a while and helped her get comfortable. I got home at 12:30 a.m. and was back at the hospital about 8:00 a.m. the next day. I tried to find out what was going on. I had a few doctors stop by and I talked to the neurologist. They just think it's a seizure, nothing more. That's an insight! I already knew that. They think it may be a reaction – an adverse reaction to her medications. Clearly, they are in the dark which doesn't make me feel confident.

Susan had seizures throughout the next day and couldn't move out of ICU to a room. The medical staff is trying to load Susan up on seizure medications so that seizures or the aura that precede the seizure(s) do not occur. No success as of this morning.

So it's Wednesday morning and here we go again. Tomorrow Matthew is being cared for by Joyce (my sister-in-law) and then Betty (my sister) on Thursday. With luck, Susan will be out of here in a few days; then back to the rehab process at home.

When will it all end? Isn't that a ridiculous question? It has only been three months since the stroke. When will it end? As the song says "we've only just begun." I'm not sure how much more she can take. This has been a real struggle. We are still trying to get organized at home and this ER event is a setback. But this too will pass and Susan will overcome. There is no other option. To think otherwise is to sell her short.

Home has been a tough struggle for Susan. She sees all that she can't do, rather than focusing on what she can do. As she pointedly informs me "tell me what I can do and I'll give it a shot." Are you supposed to be happy being unable to do basic activities like dressing? In spite of this bleak picture, Susan is happy. She is happy to be alive and is determined to figure a way out of this mess. She is tired, overwhelmed and apprehensive. This setback has devastated her confidence in being able to recover. This we will have to talk about. It is a setback not a reversal of progress. Don't I sound confident and all-knowing? It made her feel better so my little speech was worth it.

The event that sealed this decision to transfer back to Northwestern was Susan's description of an out-of-body experience. She had awakened mid afternoon on Thursday, and said "I'm going to die. I just know it." I was stunned. Not exactly the type of comment I expected to hear. "Why do you say that?" I asked. "Because I saw myself lying in bed. I was above the bed, as if on the ceiling, looking down on myself and you. I then floated out the window toward a very bright light. I could see you – see myself lying in bed, but then, even though I was lying in bed, I somehow levitated and went out the window toward the light. The light was bright and I was attracted to it. Then I woke up."

"Don't tell anyone that story or they will lock you up forever," I said, trying to make a joke and defuse the terror I felt and assumed she felt even more, especially since it was her going out the window.

"Well you are not going to die. You haven't gone through hell and back to survive and return home to all of sudden die now," I said. "We are leaving. I am calling Dr. Biller and you are going back downtown."

The nurse who was helping us (Krista) agreed with that decision. She had to call the internist, Dr. Charman to start the paperwork in support of the transfer. He agreed Susan was not getting adequate care. What bothers me, is that unless I had said "She is moving," they wouldn't have volunteered their opinion.

It was a difficult decision. You don't know if you're making "more out of this" than you should, or if there is really inadequate care going on. What if we didn't have an option? What if there was no one else to turn to for advice? We'd be screwed.

So at 4:00 in the afternoon, I began the process. I called downtown and talked to Dr. Fernandez, Dr. Biller's fellow. He said a bed could be arranged so that a transfer could take place.

I asked Krista to begin getting the ambulance at LGH so we could move downtown. She had to get the chart, the discharge orders, the medication history, and other paperwork together. It was snowing outside, and it was the rush hour.

The transport crew arrived at 6:55 p.m. and by 7:30 p.m., we were ready to roll. They would depart and I would meet them downtown. I wanted to ride along with Susan but I'd have to leave the car and I would have no way to return home.

As fate would have it, the neurologist we had been waiting to see for almost three days showed up just as Susan was being covered with blankets in preparation for the ambulance ride.

"What are you doing? What is happening?" he said. "I need to review her case and conduct a clinical exam."

I said, "Papers have been signed and we are leaving, she is extremely ill, so if I were you I would not delay us." I helped the ambulance crew get rolling by pushing the gurney.

He, the neurologist, looked stunned. Is he really surprised that we would leave after not being able to see him for almost 48 hours? He didn't say anything and just stepped aside.

We arrived at Northwestern about 8:30 p.m., not too bad given the weather (snow) and traffic. Susan was too sick to comprehend the impact of returning to the hospital where she had already lived for two months. She would not be happy being hospitalized again. But how "happy" could she have been believing she was going to die. I truly believed Susan felt she was going to die. Given that feeling, every other concern pales in comparison. Happy or not, pleased or displeased, someone has to figure out what is happening to her and do something about it.

121

We met the same old crew we knew during our first visit here about two months ago. There was Sara, Ruby and Val, all very nice and reassuring. There was an immediate sense of competence, calm, and capableness. A real feeling that the right choice was made and Susan would receive care. Nevertheless, it was an eerie feeling, like starting all over.

Susan clearly wasn't feeling well. We both were extremely anxious. In the ebb and flow of BP readings, blood draws, monitor hook-up, we reaffirmed our commitment to each other. It is "'til the end of time" and to figuring out what was going on. "You did not come all this way to allow this set-back to stand in your way. We will find out what is going on, address it so that you can get home as quickly as possible. Hang in there! There is no sense of quitting now." I said.

I think I said what I did as much for Susan as for myself. It had to be terrifying to realize you are back to square one.

I met with the resident who had instructions from Dr. Biller as to what to do. One thing they planned was a CAT scan. They wanted to see for themselves what was occurring in her brain.

I stayed until 10:00 p.m. and headed home to take care of Matthew. Betty was bringing him home, having watched him the prior night and day. I didn't know the results of the CAT scan when I left. I wanted to stay but Matthew needed me.

It was so good to see Matthew—he sort of gets lost in this shuffle. Everyone but Susan and I are taking care of him. My sister, Susan's brother, my daughters, Mother. Everyone but us. I have missed him the last couple of days. He is smiling and seems very happy. It's a great relief not to have to worry about what to do with him each and every day while Susan's health is being evaluated. Yet, at the same time, it's heartbreaking not to be able to care for him and see him change everyday. He is doing fine. I hope Susan and I can be a bigger part of his care shortly.

I got up Friday about 6:00 a.m. Matthew did real well; he slept from 11:00 p.m. until 6:00 a.m. Not bad for a little guy.

I had planned to go to work. Dora was going to watch Matthew during the day. About 8:00 a.m., Susan called and said she had talked to Dr. Biller. "You need to come downtown. He wants to talk to us sooner rather than later." The CAT scan that was done when Susan was admitted revealed a large mass. The question before us was what is the mass—an abscess or tumor? I couldn't believe I was hearing those words. This could not be starting all over again—could it?

I felt sick. I just couldn't believe what I had heard. Hell, they had done a CAT scan at Lutheran General and didn't find anything except the cloudy area that may have been blood that hadn't been reabsorbed. How could Northwestern find this mass in less than a few hours and Lutheran had been doing nothing for 3 ½ days?

Dr. Biller had been called at home and came in early because of this finding—something was seriously wrong and we had to figure out what it was. This is the type of doctor he is. He arrived early in the morning (1:00 a.m.) to look at the results of the CAT scan.

In our phone call, Susan was crying, but I said it would be fine. I would not go to work. I would come downtown directly. I called the office and Geri sounded like she was in shock as I told her what had been happening.

What to do first? There was the task of calling people, taking care of the dog, straightening up the house, starting wash, cleaning up—there are always things to do. Besides this was the heart of the morning rush. Better to get something done at home than sit in traffic.

Dora came early and she was shocked by the latest news. I told her that Amy would be coming by to help in the early afternoon as her replacement. "Don't worry," Dora said. She and everyone else had been real good about helping in whatever way they could do to relieve me of one more thing that needs to be done.

January 9 -Saturday: 4:00 p.m.

The house of cards continues to collapse around us. Susan had a brain biopsy yesterday for what they feel is an encapsulated abscess – or in terms we all can understand, a massive brain infection. I say "for what they feel" because the results are not back from pathology. The other possible explanation is a tumor— not a wonderful option. Obviously, she doesn't need the infection either, but a brain tumor this large this quick does not seem likely. If it is a brain tumor then for sure the situation is dire.

With hindsight, Susan had complained of feeling disconnected, like her head was "not all together" long before leaving rehab. I recall the car rides in which she commented that her head felt "funny," not clear. Lightheaded, feeling funny, not feeling right, difficulty concentrating, were symptoms Susan had reported more than once during the last two to three weeks of her rehab. All of these experiences were explained away as: "natural healing that takes place in the brain," "just had surgery and it takes time for everything to settle down," "perhaps it is a side effect(s) of the medications." All possible explanations which we now know were bullshit answers. No one, however, suggested a CAT scan or diagnostic studies to evaluate whether something in the brain could be causing these symptoms. It was the opinion of the medical team that nothing was going on. Only after discovering she had an infection did someone volunteer that infections rarely occur, but sadly, not rare enough for Susan. Just like a stroke rarely occurs during or after childbirth. The phrase "rarely occurs" is a clear warning that means "it will happen to us."

But, before I get along too far, let me back up and explain what has happened.

From Monday (January 4) through Thursday (January 7), Susan was in the ICU at Lutheran General Hospital with no progress being made on controlling her seizures or addressing her declining health. If anything, she was looking worse. There was almost continual vomiting, a fever, and progressive weakness. No one knew anything. The neurologist assigned to the case was no where to be found.

Having been hospitalized on a Monday, the neurologist we were assigned to did not even stop by until Wednesday, saying he was busy covering his patients and those of his partner. Busy does not appear to be a legitimate excuse for failing to see a patient in ICU for more than 36 hours. Then, when he did arrive, he did a brief exam and gave an "I'll be back shortly" response as he abruptly left the room.

I had tried to work with the doctors we were assigned, but the neurology people were incompetent. The "straw that broke the back" was the inability of the neurologist to return a page or a call from either the resident or the internist on the case. There was supposed to be an 11:00 a.m. meeting on Thursday to plan a treatment course, but it did not take place because the neurologist, Dr. Webber, failed to show up or contact me or anyone else by phone. I began to consider the possibility of Susan being transferred back to Northwestern.

The event that sealed this decision to transfer back to Northwestern was Susan's description of an out-of-body experience. She had awakened mid afternoon on Thursday, and said "I'm going to die. I just know it." I was stunned. Not exactly the type of comment I expected to hear. "Why do you say that?" I asked. "Because I saw myself lying in bed. I was above the bed, as if on the ceiling, looking down on myself and you. I then floated out the window toward a very bright light. I could see you – see myself lying in bed, but then even though I was lying in bed, I somehow levitated and went out the window toward the light. The light was bright and I was attracted to it. Then I woke up".

"Don't tell anyone that story or they will lock you up forever." I said, trying to make a joke and defuse the terror I felt and assumed she felt even more, especially since it was her going out the window – not me.

"Well you are not going to die. You haven't gone through hell and back to survive and return home to all of sudden die now." I said. "We are leaving. I am calling Biller and you are going back downtown."

Having made that decision, the nurse who was helping us (Krista) agreed. She had to call the internist, Dr. Charman to start the paperwork in support of the transfer. He agreed Susan was not getting adequate care. What bothers me is that unless I would have said "She is moving," they wouldn't have volunteered their opinion.

It was a difficult decision. You don't know if you're making "more out of this" than you should, or if there is really inadequate care going on. What if we didn't have an option? What if there was no one else to turn to for advice? We'd be screwed.

So at 4:00 in the afternoon, I began the process. I called downtown and talked to Dr. Fernandez, Dr. Biller's associate. He said a bed could be arranged so that a transfer could take place.

I asked Krista to begin getting the ambulance at LGH so we could move downtown. She had to get the chart, the discharge orders, the medication history, etc., together. In addition, it was snowing outside and it was the rush hour.

The transport crew arrived at 6:55 p.m. and by 7:30 p.m., we were ready to roll. They would depart and I would meet them downtown. I wanted to ride along with Susan but I'd have to leave the car and have no way to return home.

As fate would have it, the neurologist we had been waiting to see for almost three days showed up just as Susan was being covered with blankets in preparation for the ambulance ride.

"What are you doing? What is happening?" he said. "I need to review her case and conduct a clinical exam."

I said, "Papers have been signed and we are leaving, she is extremely ill so if I were you I would not delay us." I helped the ambulance crew get rolling by pushing the gurney.

He, the neurologist, looked stunned. Is he really surprised that we would leave after not being able to see him for almost 48 hours? He didn't say anything and just stepped aside.

We got down to Northwestern about 8:30 p.m., not too bad given the weather (snow) and traffic. Susan was too sick to comprehend the impact of returning to the hospital where she had already lived for two months. She would not be happy being hospitalized again. But how "happy" could she have been believing she was going to die. I truly believed Susan felt she was going to die. Given that feeling, every other concern pales in comparison. Happy or not, pleased or displeased, someone has to figure out what is happening to her and do something about it.

We met the same old crew we knew during our first visit here about two months ago. There was Sara, Ruby and Val, all very

126

nice and reassuring. There was an immediate sense of competence, calm, and capableness. A real feeling that the right choice was made and Susan would receive care. Nevertheless, it was an eerie feeling, like starting all over.

Susan clearly wasn't feeling well. We both were extremely anxious. In the ebb and flow of BP readings, blood draws, monitor hook-up, we reaffirmed our commitment to each other. It is "till the end of time" and to figuring out what was going on. "You did not come all this way to allow this set back to stand in your way. We will find out what is going on, address it so that you can get home as quickly as possible. Hang in there! There is no sense of quitting now." I said.

I think I said what I did as much for myself as for Susan. It had to be terrifying to realize you are back to square one.

I met with the resident who had instructions from Dr. Biller as to what to do. One thing they planned was a CAT scan. They wanted to see for themselves what was occurring in her brain.

I stayed until 10:00 p.m. and headed home to take care of Matthew. Betty was bringing him home, having watched him the prior night and day. I didn't know the results of the CAT scan when I left. I wanted to stay but Matthew needed me.

It was so good to see Matthew—he sort of gets lost in this shuffle. Everyone but Susan and I are taking care of him. My sister, Susan's brother, my daughters, mother. Everyone but us. I have missed him the last couple of days. He is smiling and seems very happy. It's a great relief not to have to worry about what to do with him each and every day, while Susan's health is being evaluated. Yet, at the same time, it's heartbreaking not to be able to care for him and see him change everyday. He is doing fine. I hope Susan and I can be a bigger part of his care shortly.

I got up Friday about 6:00 a.m. Matthew did real well; he slept from 11:00 p.m. until 6:00 a.m. Not bad for a little guy.

I had planned to go to work. Dora was going to watch Matthew during the day. About 8:00 a.m., Susan called and said she had talked to Dr. Biller. "You need to come downtown. He wants to talk to us sooner rather than later." At 1:00 a.m., Dr. Biller came to the hospital to review the CAT scan that was done when she was admitted. The CAT scan revealed a large mass. The question before us is what is the mass—an abscess or tumor? I couldn't believe I was hearing those words. This could not be starting all over again—could it?

I felt sick. I just couldn't believe what I had heard. Hell, they had done a CAT scan at Lutheran General and didn't find anything except the cloudy area that may have been blood that hadn't been reabsorbed. How could Northwestern find this mass in less than a few hours and Lutheran had been doing nothing for 3 and a half days?

Dr. Biller had been called at home and came in early because of this finding—something was seriously wrong and we had to figure out what it was. This is the type of doctor he is. He arrived early in the morning (1:00am) to personally look at the results of the CAT scan.

In our phone call, Susan was crying, but I said it would be fine. I would not go to work. I would come downtown directly. I called the office and Geri sounded like she was in shock as I told her what had been happening.

What to do first? There was the task of calling people, taking care of the dog, straightening up the house, starting wash, cleaning up—there are always things to do. Besides this was the heart of the morning rush. Rather get something done at home than sit in traffic.

Dora came early and she was shocked by the latest news. I told her that Amy would be coming by to help in the early afternoon as her replacement. "Don't worry"—she and everyone else had been real good about helping in whatever way they can each relieving me of one more thing that had to be done.

January 12 - Tuesday: 10:00 a.m.

Never any time to finish telling the story; things always happen. It's now Tuesday and I am trying to talk about what occurred last Friday. Let me go back and finish the story and try to get us up to date.

Last Friday I went downtown because Susan had talked to Dr. Biller, who said there was a mass in her head, either a tumor or an abscess (infection)—either way it wasn't good. I was stunned as she told me "abscess/tumor." How much more can she take? It's not like she didn't have enough to deal with.

"I'll be right down." I was going to go into work and get back in the swing of things. This week had been a vacation week. What a joke! We had planned to do a lot of things around the house, but the seizures and hospitalization altered our plans.

As I got ready, all I could think about is "here we go again." A little more than two months ago Susan had had the brain surgery and was eventually transferred to this same room. Now we are back in the same hospital/same room again. It could not be a tumor—she just couldn't have surgery. Not again.

It was 9:00 a.m. and I headed downtown. Traffic wasn't too bad, although it was heavy in spots. When I arrived, I had a very uncomfortable feeling walking around the hospital's grounds, the buildings, the halls where we had been and are now back again.

I'd see nurses, doctors, transportation aides who I either know or recognize. Sort of scary when you remember their names and they remember you. Shows you how long Susan had been hospitalized. To be remembered by the transportation staff says it all.

I got to Susan's room and she looked very sick and terrified. Who wouldn't? She had 50,000 questions and no answers. Questions without answers caused anxiety. Left to her own conclusions, the answers she'd come up with would always be the worst outcome. Of course, why would it be a positive outcome? What is positive about the past two months? Sounds bitter. Sounds angry. Sounds scared. Should I, we, sound any different?

Susan was concerned she had a tumor and that brain surgery would be necessary to correct the problem. This is the first time I began to see a major crack in her confidence and hope. What she had been through and what she was trying to cope with were more than anyone should have to confront. Now she has another hospitalization, perhaps impending surgery, and in all likelihood, a return trip to rehab. Susan was devastated. She was only home for a few days and then re-institutionalized/re-hospitalized. Not a good start to the new year. So much for our optimistic outlook for 1993.

My style is to make fun of the pain I am feeling. To do otherwise is to be consumed by the pain. Like the old adage "Laugh and the world laughs with you; weep and you weep alone." The more anxious she looked, the more I'd say, "At least you're not anxious." It was clear to me that this round of trouble had affected her more psychologically than the first round of trouble. She knew more about what was at stake. What might have to be done. What could go wrong. You could see it in her face—the uncertainty, the anxiety, the fear. It had caught her and I knew it.

I tried to reassure her that "things will be fine." What else can you say? To say it will be ok sounds stupid, because what do I know about abscesses or tumors? Yet, it needs to be said to give some reassurance, some hope that as someone once said, "This too shall pass." You just have to say, and more importantly believe, that "things will be ok." There is really no sense of thinking otherwise. To do so admits defeat and resignation, and Susan had not survived all she had been through to begin to think negativlye.

I arrived while Dr. Biller was entering Susan's room – perfect timing.

"Good morning! Glad you could come down early. I was about to explain things to Susan, so we can have this conversation all together.r" He continued, *"I told Susan last night that the CAT scan revealed a large mass in the brain at the site of the surgery. We don't know what it is and we really need to know."*

"What do you think it is?" I asked.

"It is either a tumor, which Susan grew overnight, something I don't believe it is or it is an encapsulated abscess or infection which seeded in the brain following surgery. I think it is an infection and we have to do a sterostactic biopsy to determine the nature of the infection."

Susan and I said nothing and continued listening.

> *Dr. Biller continued, "If it is an infection that has a hard shell to it (encapsulated) we have to obtain a sample of the matter so we can grow it, culture it, and decide how to treat it. This infection, let us assume that is what it is, has to be treated with drugs, surgery is really not an option, given where it is and what tissue would have to be removed to get at it. Too much good tissue would be affected. You would lose functional and cognitive abilities to such an extent that it would be unacceptable.*

I translated this to mean that Susan would be substantially paralyzed and perhaps with little cognitive ability, but the infection would have been removed.

> *"So what do you plan to do?" Susan asked.*

> *"We obtain a sample of the mass, culture it in order to identify what medication to use. If that doesn't work, meaning we can't identify a specific bacteria, then I would recommend a course of massive amounts of broad spectrum antibiotics to try and kill it, resolve it, and this could take eight to ten weeks of intensive medication treatment."*

I couldn't believe all the possible complications—bleed, tumor, infection—again, not knowing made things more difficult because we weren't sure what we were facing or what we had to deal with. Dr. Biller seemed convinced it was an infection because he did not know of any condition that would allow a tumor to grow as fast and as large as this mass had become.

I went over to rehab to talk with Dr. Smith about Susan's readmission. Dr. Smith couldn't believe it either. My goodness, who the hell can? Make up the wildest story or series of events you can and it doesn't even approach what Susan has encountered. As Dr. Smith and I talked, a call came in for me. Dr. Biller said the neurosurgeons wanted to do the surgery **now**. The doctor was available. Could I hurry back to her room. The sooner something definitive was known as to what this mass was, the sooner plans could be made to do something about it.

My heart dropped. While I knew surgery was likely and at some time during the day, it didn't dawn on me that it would be now—right now. I rushed back to Susan's room to meet the surgeon.

Dr. Levy, who specializes in this type of procedure, was going to operate. There is a technical name for the procedure (sterostactic biopsy), but the simplest way to comprehend it is to consider it brain surgery. It's a surgical procedure; it is just not as major as the evacuation she had two months ago, but then again that is easy for me to say. I'm not sure I'd be so cavalier if a steel halo was being screwed onto my head to act as a guide for drilling into my brain. That's right. Drilling!

Now listen to me talk. Not major—any time they do something in the head, it's major/big time. Cleaning teeth is major to me. Compared to what Susan had already experienced, this procedure was relatively minor.

Dr. Levy, a pleasant man, described what he would do, how it would be done, and how long the procedure would take. Susan and I didn't need to hear about the possible complications like a stroke, another bleed, or all the other problems we didn't want to hear, but he ran through the list, and as best as we could, we ignored the information. The biopsy had to be done and this approach was certainly preferred to either doing nothing or another craniotomy.

I signed the consent forms and Dr. Levy and his group of associates began the process of drawing blood, doing an EKG, booking the OR, etc. It is not as easy as you think—going for surgery takes a lot of effort and cooperation on the part of many individuals.

By 1:30 p.m., transportation had arrived and Susan was ready to go. She started to cry. She wanted to say goodbye, like this was the end. I could not tolerate it. As always, I made a joke and went along in a mocking way. I could not do this seriously. That would be too painful and reinforce the perception of the problem being extremely serious. "How do you think I feel having to sit and wait? At least you know what they are doing. Don't forget 'only the good die young' and you are too old for that to happen." Jokes that made neither of us laugh. Finally, before she left the room on the cart, I said, "I will see you when they are done. I will be right outside the door waiting for you and I'll give you a kiss." She smiled as best as she could. "Better be ready for the kiss," she said. With that Susan was wheeled out of the room and off to the OR.

Susan's mother and dad just happened to be visiting. They had planned to see Susan not knowing anything about the day's events. Rather than wait to find out the results of surgery, Otto, Susan's father decided to leave so he could beat the traffic. Otto doesn't know what to say or do—so he leaves. That's okay, because it's one less thing to worry about – or deal with.

Susan's mother. Viola, stayed and went with us as we rolled over to Olsen (the building in which the operation will be done) for the start of surgery. The first thing that had to be done was to bolt this metal crown to her head to guide the markings they'd make from the CAT scan. While it didn't take long (15 minutes) to put into place, it looked terrible. She looked like she had been in a car accident and had this halo to wear in order to stabilize her neck and head.

I went with her and stayed with her while the CAT scan was done. This picture with the halo allows the surgeon to figure out where the mass is. You don't want to shove needles blindly into the head. There is no telling what you'd hit. Susan didn't want to have any further trouble. It was bad enough that she had to go through this procedure two months post-surgery. So it is best to get things done correctly to minimize any possibility of error.

I walked along the side of her cart back to the OR room. The medical staff allowed me to wait with her until the surgeon was ready to do the procedure. I left in a few minutes and took her mom to get something to eat. By this time, it was 5:00 p.m. and the process of getting ready for the surgery had already consumed 3½ hours.

The biopsy itself would take only a half hour. It was done under local anesthetic. Can you believe that? The specimen Dr. Levy obtained would be examined immediately to decide whether enough had been acquired so that a determination as to the type of infection could be made. If so, the surgery was over and all we had to do was wait for the cultures to grow.

Susan's hair was coming back in, until they shaved another 2x5 inch patch within the initial surgical area. The biopsy was taken from within the original surgical boundaries.

I waited with her mother and Carole, her niece. Carole had come by after work. Carole was very upset to learn about the surgery. There was nothing she or Susan's mother could do. Nothing any of us could do except wait.

Dr. Levy came down around six to tell us that everything points to an infection. Susan tolerated the surgery well, the procedure itself went fine, and she was ready to return to her room. I was waiting for her when she was wheeled out of the OR. As we saw each other she asked, "Where is that kiss you promised?"

January 14 - Thursday: 5:02 p.m.
Let me provide an update on what has been occurring. Susan did well following surgery. She has been very tired and weak. Vomiting occurred, but it is all part of the head trauma— seizures and what has been defined as a massive infection at the site of the original bleed/surgery.

Since last Friday we have been waiting for the biopsy results. The objective is to know the bug, so you can give the right drug. Well as easy as that sounds, it hasn't been easy. Because she had been started on antibiotics when she was admitted, the very infection we are attempting to type may be changing as a result of treatment, thus impacting the ability to culture it.

For the last four to five days we have not known what type of infection it is and that makes the ability to plan a course of treatment impossible. The real concern is how long she will be in the hospital. We have been told everything from, "she'll be going home Thursday (today)," to "she'll be here four to six weeks." Keep in mind, Dr. Biller had said 8 – 10 weeks. Such a span of time makes it hard to plan. Susan was planning on staying the least amount of time.

Helping with Matthew, again, is beating up my mom and Dora. They have returned for their second tour of duty. After three months, both have had enough. My mother has to get her health back and prepare for her previously planned upcoming cruise; I know she'll love it. Dora just has to get on with her life—enough is enough. I have to get some order and stability, so I do not have to worry about who will be taking care of Matthew.

I will try and take Tom McCabe, a colleague at work, up on his offer to share baby-sitters for awhile, until Susan comes home and I can figure out what arrangements she needs. I'm going to talk to Mrs. McCabe today and plan to have Matthew stay with her on Monday. I'll still have him, the house, and the rest when I come home from work, but that's the way it is. This way he can have a daycare outing while I am at work. Mrs. McCabe recently had a baby and already has help. Matthew will simply be joining the group.

The last few days, I have begun to feel overwhelmed. The sheer responsibility for everything is oppressive. Three months has been a long time and the days seem like they are getting longer. This is especially true with this last hospitalization. I just couldn't believe there was this issue confronting us again (brain surgery). Never in my wildest dreams did I think this would occur. Why would anyone think anything else could happen after all that has already happened? Because of Susan's situation and limitations, I am practically a single parent—a Mr. Mom. Ninety-five percent of the time that is not a big deal. But when I get tired, or Matthew doesn't cooperate (as if he has a choice), it becomes a real struggle. I just want to lie down and have quiet time. Forget about fun or exercising or doing anything I'd like to do. For me, right now, quiet and some sleep are all I need.

The job, Susan, and Matthew—consume the day and night. All three take effort. I'll give you an example. A few days ago, I had just finished feeding Matthew at 6:30 a.m., started to sit down so I wouldn't fall over, and Hans, our dog, started vomiting. He and I were outside so he could throw up, barefoot of course, since I had no chance to put on shoes. When I came in, Matthew was crying. And, of course, since Matthew was crying, Hans started to bark like he had to go to the bathroom, which he really did because we didn't take any time for him to do his business when we were out there earlier.

You can tell, my penmanship (I wrote this book in long-hand) is not real clear—that is simply because I am falling asleep as I write this.

Susan's mood could be better, but it also could be much worse. She is very disgusted and depressed about "everything." I told her not to say depressed, because they'll order a psych consult which is all she needs; then, for sure, Susan will never leave the place or return home. Dysphoric sounds better.

Matthew awoke at 4:10 a.m. and I decided to stay up. It is "quiet time" because my mother is sleeping. No one else is up. Nobody is calling on the phone—sort of the best time. Never thought "4:10 a.m." would be the "best time" ever!

So here I continue to sit at 5:40 a.m. Hans has to be walked; dishes done; clothes washed; house picked up; driveway shoveled; a few bills paid; and, this is just the start of a typical day.

Dr. Biller will be in today, so we are hoping to find out the treatment plan – the only component of interest is when Susan will be coming home.

Susan sounded very disgusted last night, so in spite of feeling exhausted, I decided to pick up Matthew and head downtown with my mother. Susan was very surprised and extremely happy. I knew seeing Matthew would help her spirits and it did. She just wants to be a mom, be who she was – all reasonable requests which are becoming exceedingly hard to fulfill.

We stayed for 1½ hours. I had to get back with Matthew because he has a schedule. He was good and Susan was shocked at how much he had grown in just a week.

Matthew had a little spit-up and diarrhea. I hope he isn't getting anything or picked up something from the hospital. I don't think that happened.

Well I have had a 50-minute break, so it's time to move on for another day of fun.

January 17 - Sunday: 10:45 p.m.

Tears come easy for Susan, and why not. She is aware of the struggle she has waged to get to where she is and now she is faced with an extra load of uncertainty. It's bad enough not to be sure and certain of what will happen. When all hell breaks loose, it confirms the deep fear you have had and now you're faced with the uncertainty again, only magnified. However, this new trouble has reinforced Susan's belief that shit can and does happen (things can get worse). Therefore, how hopeful can she allow herself to be?

I have tried to support her by being sarcastic when she gets down. Acknowledging the legitimacy of her fears/feelings, but trying to get her to move beyond them. Sort of kick in the ass and pat on the back all at the same time. I have to give her credit – once she expresses her frustration her next comment is "how are you?" This is her gift - says what is on her mind and then expresses concern for someone else. Regardless of her predicament, Susan is much more concerned about others than herself.

I went to work Friday; Dora and Amy watched Matthew. Work was okay, but my mind is not there. I have enough trouble focusing on what I like and want to do, let alone all that shit about quality control and quality teams, etc., that the work-site is pushing. It's a waste of time and energy and really diverts us from what we have to do—rebuild the treatment services.

Amy stayed with Matthew until I got home, then it was he and I (plus Hans) Friday night. Matthew is fine. He has gas and is fussy at times, but overall he does well.

I was able to "sleep" Friday night - not that much, sort of 4-hour stretches. Matthew did well—sleeping and eating. We got up early Saturday and ran around doing chores. Wherever I go, he goes. We ran a few errands (groceries, hardware store, bank, etc.). He goes along for the ride and loves it.

Betty and John came by in the afternoon. Matthew was spending the day and an overnight at their place. I took care of Hans, picked up the house and got cleaned up. I was heading downtown to spend the day with Susan.

I know I've complained about this before, but the lack of time to do anything, plus the lack of time to do what I want to do for myself (although when pressed I have no answer for the question "what do I want to do," perhaps it is best to quit bringing this up) is overwhelming. It's like choices and options have disappeared from my life. I listen to what other people have to say about their plans and suggestions, and go along with them. There really are no choices or options; things have to get done or taken care of and I do them. Simple as that. It is best to keep it simple – complaining, although I do my fair share (to myself of course) wastes time and accomplishes nothing. I just shut-up and move on. It doesn't take much to realize that my issues pale in comparison to what Susan confronts.

A good example is washing clothes. I'm suppose to let them pile up and then, once a week, someone can come over and do them. In principle that sounds okay, but I can throw in one or two loads a day and do them overnight. That is just as easy, because at least I can have a say over the clothes I want to wear. Any small measure of control is huge.

How long will Susan stay in the hospital? That is the burning question. We all want it to be short, but we all think (and won't say) that it will be long (four to six weeks). The problem is the extent and seriousness of the infection and the need to have IV fluids/antibiotics directly for at least three weeks, which doesn't count the rehab time that will be necessary to get Susan back on her feet. Susan will have to do rehab to give her the best chance of returning to baseline.

Not to give herself this chance is short-changing herself. The bind is the length of time she will need to be in the hospital. This new stretch is on top of the time she has already spent away. All this time away is time away from Matthew. Collectively, these events make any time in the hospital unthinkable. Matthew's growing, changing, and doing things. She is not there to be a part of it and these lost experiences are killing her. No matter how she and I try to put things in context and attempt to make sense of the situation, or to rationally comprehend it, Matthew doesn't have Mommy, and Mommy doesn't have Matthew. That is it in a nutshell. It is even simpler: Susan can't care for Matthew. She can't even do the basic things for him because she has physical limitations and can't even do some of the basics for herself. Once she begins to feel better and stronger on her left side, she should be able to help out more. Then the problem is Matthew. He is going to become mobile and she won't be able to keep up with him. So there is always going to be this disjuncture in her ability to truly feel like his Mom. But doing things for a child is not the only way to be a Mom. Being there to teach, talk with, offer advice, be a confidant, be an example of strength and character. These Susan can do and in due time she will feel like his Mom. These changes will occur over time. We will have to wait and see. No one should mistake the fact that Susan is the Mom, a capable Mom who needs some assistance.

Dr. Smith is looking into a bed at rehab. The debate between Dr. Biller, Susan and Dr. Smith is about whether Susan is medically stable enough to go to rehab. Are there more tests to do and is the infection under control and shrinking? If this doesn't happen, forget rehab because we're talking more surgery; so the first priority is the infection and reducing the abscess. When this occurs, Susan will be medically cleared and the road home goes through rehab.

I spent most of yesterday downtown. Susan had visitors throughout the day: the Mayers (friends of ours) and Beth (one of Susan's best friends). I came about 3:00 p.m. and Jim and Carole came about 6:00 p.m. I left about 9:00 p.m. It was a full day and a good day for Susan because she was occupied during most of the day. There was no time to think about or dwell on what she was missing at home.

I ordered a "room service" meal like I did for our anniversary. Susan wanted crab cakes and that was a good way to encourage her to eat. She had a good dinner: crab cakes, salad, ice cream and bread. At least, she is eating. The staff is worried Susan is not eating enough. Her protein level is low and this will not help her fight infection. Dr. Biller told us to bring food from home, or whatever it takes for her to eat and regain her strength.

I am worried about her mood. She is getting beaten up by all the testing, possible surgery talk, doubts about what functioning will return, and missing Matthew. Collectively it is all taking a toll.

I hope she can weather this, in addition to everything else. She will, there is no choice. Now is not the time to quit. If Susan wanted to quit, she should have done it earlier; she would have saved us all a lot of time. Thank God Susan didn't quit, so now is not the time to think about that. There is far too much living ahead that we will enjoy. I need her to be my partner in this journey.

We have invested too much into getting our lives back to quit now. Stopping or quitting is not an option. Like myself, Susan can pause, have a bad moment, but we must move forward. Forward is the only way to go.

January 18 - Monday: 6:30 p.m.

I just looked at the clock. It is only 6:30 p.m. and it feels like midnight. Today "day care" for Matthew began. I drop him off before work and pick him up on the way home. Something different for the both of us. This was day one of doing it all by myself and, if this day is typical (which I hope it isn't), it will be a long, long haul until some sense of normalcy returns. I sometimes wonder if that is just a hope. Will there ever be anything like it was before? I don't know. With the baby, it certainly won't, but like I said this is only day one and maybe the rest will be different.

Interesting how I keep trying to look on the bright side of things. What else can you do? You can stop looking for the bright side, but why would you? It takes a lot of energy to be upbeat and buoyant. Realistically, there is no choice in my mind but to be upbeat, but it is difficult at times. While I give myself this pep talk, what must Susan do to remain positive in spite of her moments, and we all have them. She is extremely positive. This is a source of strength for me.

Based on the conversations I have had with Drs. Biller and Smith, I'd say four to six weeks of hospitalization at a minimum is what Susan is facing. This infection is no joke and the only real way to treat it is with massive amounts of broad based antibiotics via an IV. They put a line into her chest wall so they can easily accomplish this task. Since they can't identify the specific type of infection she has, the culture did not reveal this, then the only thing to do is throw everything at it and hope something sticks. If this approach doesn't work then surgery will most surely be required.

There is no quick fix—it's that simple—so on we go.

Matthew got up at 11:45 p.m. and 4:00 a.m. I've been up since 3:30 a.m. and won't get to bed until 10:00 p.m. (a 19 hour day). Just getting things organized and packed and put into the car, plus him and me is at least an hour to an-hour-and-a-half project. Then you have to unpack him, explain the rules to the caregiver, and then go on the way to work. I'm beginning to realize what people go through to keep to this schedule. At least with a timetable that has to be met, everyone is focused. Then there is the dog, he wants attention or to go outside for a walk. Seems reasonable for me. I will have to figure who can do this while I am away for long periods during the day.

I start to get organized the night before the next day; that's the only way. In the morning I just do what has to be done; there is no time to remember anything; the less I have to think about, the better. It's just impossible to think. The morning is for doing things, not thinking about what to do!

I got up at 3:30, stayed up, and fed Matthew around 4:15 a.m. By the time he was finished, it was almost 5:00 a.m. and there was no sense in going back to bed. I did wash (always wash) and picked up around the house. I got dressed so I'd be ready when he got up. That was a mistake. While I was changing him, he peed on my suit so I had to change my clothes after he was dressed. I quickly learned the importance of strategically placing a towel on him while dressing him.

I finally got on the way about 7:30 a.m. and got to Tom's house (the babysitter's place) and met everybody: his wife, child, new son and the sitter. I felt funny leaving him at their home; but there is no choice. Like a lot of things in my life right now, there are no choices. You would think having no choices would simplify things but it hasn't as of yet. Having choices gives one a sense of control, a feeling that I, and I am sure Susan, would dearly love to have.

Work was uneventful. I caught up on mail and calls and finally finished a draft of a research paper. Made appointments; scheduled meetings; tried to get work and our personal activities on track. Talked with Susan a few times to try and keep her spirits up. She is depressed and heading south. Both she and I know it. The last thing we need is for her to get depressed. Who the hell is real happy anyway? Be sad, don't be depressed. Complain and move on. I can only imagine how hard it must be for Susan to find the strength and the will to move on – yet she always does. Thank God!

Now is not the time to quit. So it's a long haul. She has been through too much to turn around now. It would be crazy to do so. She knows it, but the hospital stay and being away from home are becoming oppressive for her. The meaning and sources of joy in her life are absent: she is not home; not with Matthew, me or the dog. Susan is not who she was. It is not only her health, but missing Matthew that weighs on her. These collective concerns, along with this new hospitalization, the uncertainty about the brain abscess all resulting in a new sense of doom and gloom. It is not a positive mental state. But so what! I'm not going to quit. Neither will she.

I think Susan finally realizes how serious the infection is. If the infection cannot be resolved through medications, then it's surgery and possibly her life. Why she hadn't caught on to the scope of the problem before is beyond me, but I think she does now. Perhaps she can't allow herself to consider the moment. Denial is a useful strategy. Whatever the source of these depressive feelings, they will pass because I know Susan. She is determined to do whatever she has to do to get back with us at home.

What Susan doesn't like is the prospect of three to six weeks of hospital time facing her and the non-use of her left side which she had managed to regain some function on before this setback. No doubt this is a setback due to the seizures and now the infection, but all that can be regained and then some. I just feel she is really uncertain about the future, given the turn of events that have happened. Who can blame her? It's not as if I am all-knowing and can predict the future. The next few moments are as far ahead as I can go myself.

Therein lies the dilemma—being optimistic in the face of bad news. There has to be some reality for the optimism to grow. Hope needs to be reinforced somehow – someway. One needs specific concrete signs of progress in order to continue to be hopeful. Miracles have already occurred; she survived, is herself, and can get better. It's how quickly can "I get my old self back" that is the bind. In all honesty her and our lives ended with these events, we are now about building a new life – just how that is supposed to happen is unclear – or should I say uncertain.

I was planning to wear a suit tomorrow, but my only pair of shoes has the sole come loose. I'm trying to glue them now. I will have to wait and see if it works. I might have to stop on the way to work and buy a pair of shoes.

Since picking Matthew up on the way home at 3:45 p.m. he has been screaming and crying; perhaps these are tears of joy that I have returned. I sure hope so. If I am correct, he can quiet down knowing I am now here. Matthew has a hard time burping and consequently develops gas and spits up. So all he has been doing for the last 2½ hours is yelling. He is hoarse; no matter what I do it doesn't work. He will have to cry himself to sleep. After three hours, I have had enough. I'm going to sleep whether he wants me to or not.

Let's see what tomorrow holds.

Susan and I wanted to do something special for Dr. Biller's birthday so we bought a birthday cake and pulled off a surprise impromptu celebration. The surprise party really went well. He appreciated it very much. He was embarrassed, so it was a success. I'm not sure any patient he has had in the past planned a surprise birthday party for him while he was making rounds. But this is Susan, she is the party girl and wanted to acknowledge his birthday in a special way.

I fell asleep for 1½ hours and awoke to hear Matthew continuing to cry. So we are going on five hours. I guess he is stubborn. I fed him his bottle and he is now smiling in his chair. Maybe he was hungry all this time. I need to get on the ball and find out when he last ate when I pick him up from the sitter. Sort of stupid on my part not to think of food.

January 21 - Thursday: 5:25 a.m.

To say that I have gotten accustomed to all this is not exactly the whole story. It's more correct to say I just do what I can, as I can, when I can. I now conform to Matthew's schedule—how dumb to think he'd fit into my obligations and timetable. This obviously shows great adaptability on my part.

The best news we had in a long time was that the CAT scan done today revealed the abscess has begun to shrink, an indication that the antibiotics are working. Everyone except Dr. Biller recommended surgery, but it is no longer a consideration. He chose to be cautious; he knew the antibiotic would eventually do the job and it seems to have paid off.

Susan's spirits are much better. At least things are moving along and they are going in the right direction. She has been very depressed with "everything," and in this case, "everything" is perfectly clear. **EVERYTHING!** It isn't just this or that—it's everything! Funny to say this, but I know what she means when she says everything. Everything actually covers everything quite well.

The CAT scan news and visits by Matthew are helping her get through this second hospitalization. But the visits by Matthew are still painful. She can hold him in her lap, feed him if he is propped up, but that's about it. Playing with him on her shoulder; changing his clothes/diapers; trying to comfort him; repositioning him in her arms or up on her shoulder—these actions are just impossible. Seeing me do these things (enjoying him) makes the missing out even more painful. Watching Matthew be joyful is not the same as being the source of his joy.

Every time she sees Matthew, she comments on how much he has grown. Well you can imagine all that is missed between the growth spurts. Wanting/wishing to do things, and being unable to, is very difficult for her. The more I enjoy him, the more she knows how much she has missed. It's true; that's reality; and, perhaps it can be corrected or changed in the near future. But right now it still sucks.

Work, Matthew, house, Susan, Hans (plus whatever else) have been an absolute whirlwind. Aside from brief moments of quiet or silence or just "moments to catch my breath," it's non-stop. Matthew takes between an hour and a half and two hours to get up, fed, cleaned up, dressed, readied to leave the house, packed and placed in the car, plus me trying to get ready and just put the house back into some order after I walk the dog.

Then we drive. I cart him into the babysitter's and then resume my trip. Repeat the cycle coming home and then continue the chores that need to be done (cook, Hans, garbage, laundry, etc.) between feedings, clothes changes, crying, phone calls. Believe it or not, this is not an exhaustive list—just "off the top of my head responsibilities." This is what it is and since I am keeping up with it, this schedule of activities is probably not as demanding as I make it out to be.

Susan was moved to another bed; same floor, but less intense than acute intensive care. I think she has resigned to being there three to five weeks—not all at once, but daily. As she said last night, "I don't know how I'll last another day," but then she does and resumes the challenge of getting through another day. You can only go a mile one step at a time. Susan has this remarkable ability to just keep at it. She has a resolve and determination that knows no limits. There is no "quit" in her.

Matthew and I paid a surprise visit to Susan. She loved it. To say she "lives for it" would not be an understatement. Susan fed and played with Matthew and got to show him off to the nurses and doctors. We had a short, but fun visit, but the tears and pain are always there. That's just the way it is.

I'm staying home this morning. I will go downtown later in the day to be with Susan. Matthew's big sisters will watch him. I will pick up the house and get things together for the weekend.

January 23 - Saturday: 8:20 p.m.

Depression! That is the operative word. Not that she hasn't felt profoundly sad before. But this time the ability to bounce back emotionally is missing. For the last week or so, Susan has begun to experience a deep sadness. Who wouldn't? Like it's a surprise! But it is clearly depression and it is leaving a marked impact on her. She is quiet. No real affect. Fewer questions about Matthew, me, anything.

We have talked about this. She is able to express her feelings to me, to her friends Beth, Melinda—so she is able to talk and cry about things. That's about all that she can do. What will a psychologist/psychiatrist do? Process feelings? What a bunch of shit. At some point the emotional weight of these events is suffocating. Somehow she is going to have to catch a second wind. She will.

Dr. Fernandez, a colleague of Dr. Biller, characterized Susan's state: "It's an acute depression, explainable by what has occurred over the past three months." It's as simple or as complicated as that. He told Susan she has to get on with life. She can't lie in bed (never has). She has to get her ass up and shower, clean up (always does). Now is not the time to feel sorry for herself (not that she ever has). How does she, me, we, get on with life is unclear. Let's just say it is far easier for Fernandez to say "get on with life" than it is to try and do it. Nevertheless, it sounds like we should be doing things. Taking action is the strategy for attacking depression. Do more and you will feel better. Of course, what do I know. Probably as much as any of these other so-called experts. I don't know how anyone can survive, physically and emotionally, what Susan has experienced. That she has survived is a miracle and a testament to her tremendous personal strength.

I had a good meeting at work with my colleagues David, Jean, and Anita. The rest of the company is a joke, but we will move on and survive. I'm going to Wisconsin on Wednesday to work out the contract details on the study the Wisconsin alcohol providers want us to do. I will also meet with another company on Thursday; things will start to break.

Matthew had a doctor's visit. He is doing great (9 lbs., 6 oz. and 22" long). Things couldn't be better for him (aside from having Mom home which is a huge aside) and the day care sitter is working out well. Thanks be to God for small favors. Matthew received a few shots at the doctor's today so he might be cranky and run a fever; should be a fun night.

Susan was crying this morning (while I'm up to my ass in ten projects, before I leave to go to the pediatrician). I told her I had to get going. She was put off, but I explained that I had things to do and we'd talk later.

It got ironed out; she just needed to talk and, as I explained, I just needed to get things done in order to come down and see her, which I did, and pick Grandma up on the way back. Any kind of break would be okay with me. This has been a long haul for all of us. The word nightmare gives only a flavor of the terror and pain.

Susan looked good, but is bothered by a low-grade fever and her hand shakes. I think it is drug related. The seizure medication is causing some of this, plus her depression/anxiety doesn't help any. At any moment, she is ready to jump out of her skin. Then she is confronted by the four walls day in and day out. That's enough to drive anyone crazy. Susan has a lot of time to think about what has happened; what she can't do and/or won't do, and together, that's enough to drive her nuts. How can you not be obsessed, review and be preoccupied during every waking moment with what has happened? To not would be crazy.

Two nurses from rehab (Joanna and Renee) came by to see her. That was very nice of them to use their break to come over and say, Hi!

Jim and Carole also visited, and that helped pass the time. I've already talked with Susan a couple of times tonight. So the evening has passed fairly well and I'll be heading downtown tomorrow (but without Matthew). Matthew may not be up to par tomorrow, we'll see. Also, I don't want him to catch anything at the hospital and get sick.

He is down for the night. He ate and I gave him aspirin, and he is out until about 1:00 a.m. I hope there are no real problems as a result of the shots.

I stopped on the way home from the hospital to get a pizza and fell asleep waiting for it to be made. The waitress had to wake me up as I had my head down on the counter. That's scary; at the drop of a hat I can sleep.

I'm gaining weight and will have to try and start exercising or something, like maybe shut my mouth so the food doesn't get in in the first place. Exercise would help with the weight and help burn off steam. Maybe I'll try running tomorrow.

Well I'm off to the basement for more wash, then a nap (this is what I refer to as my night's sleep, a nap, because by the time I am in bed – 11:00 pm – and Matthew is up – 3:00 am or 4:00 am all I have been able to get is a nap) before I get up for the early morning feeding.

January 28 - Thursday: 4:50 a.m.

Matthew got up about 4:00 a.m. and did well in the sense that he slept from about 10:00 p.m.

I went to Madison, Wisconsin yesterday to present outcome stuff—long day, long ride, but it is a contract so that's what counts.

Susan is making concrete progress. Walking more, even though she sees herself as "having a long way to go," instead of "I've come a long way already." Both are true, but at times she is short to give herself credit for what she has been able to accomplish. It is a huge accomplishment to have lived – walking is a miracle.

I'm trying to work, get Matthew organized, and see Susan, let alone take care of the house and chores. Needless to say, it doesn't all get done. At times, it is overwhelming (what a broken record). I'd like to sit and not have to think or do anything—that's what I would like to do. But that option is not readily available at this time. To be honest, I can't even think of anything that I'd like to do. Not a good sign.

I noticed how much easier it was to have Matthew stay at home and have Mother (later Dora) help, rather than pack him up and head out to day care. Obviously, it's easier. Someone else helping is a help!

Where Susan is at in her current hospital stay is unclear. How things get confused is beyond me. The problem is the transfer from Dr. Biller (Neurology) to Dr. Smith (Rehab). The linkage, planning and coordination is not there. So the options run the gamut of leaving the hospital with no need for rehab versus transfer Friday to rehab for a week to ten days of rework prior to going home. Since there is so much to get organized and coordinated, it seems the best is to move on to rehab—but smoothly. Dr. Smith is checking on a bed.

Susan, obviously and rightly wants out—now! Who can blame her? Yet is she ready? What about home care; the IV's; the rehab appointments? There are other critical questions that need to be resolved, plus set up home care arrangements.

We are leaving the hospital after three weeks or so rather than three to six weeks in the hospital. Rehab will follow. I was able to convince our insurance company that paying a shorter inpatient stay and adding some outpatient services to cover the nurses, PT, OT and whatever else is needed at home is saving them (the insurance company) money and allowing us to get to rehab and home quicker.

It is a win-win for all parties. Something tells me I should have received this "agreement" in writing to document this adjustment in benefits, before adjusting the length of inpatient stay. In some ways it doesn't matter, Susan wants out at any cost. However, to have the availability (in writing) of additional outpatient services above the allotted number would have been smart. Somehow, I don't really think the insurance company would have provided a letter.

The central line will stay in her chest and that is how she will receive her antibiotic treatments at home. It will have to be kept clean, but that should be relatively straightforward. Home is a much better place to receive the medicine than in the hospital.

So we are all in agreement – the road home goes through rehab, the sooner we get there for a refresher course, the better, and then home again.

All this points to the issue of control or the lack of it in our lives. Neither Susan nor I has a say in this process. Since it (the outcome of whatever is decided) chiefly affects us, you'd hope we'd be intimately involved in what's being decided. Well, it hasn't happened and this is frustrating. I will make sure all the principals are on the same page so we can move on, and then on to home.

I have meetings downtown today, so I'm going to see Susan both before and after the meetings. We are unable to spend any time alone because I can't visit as often and when I do, Matthew is along and we try and do as much as we can with him, plus keep him happy. So it's not easy to visit and take care of Matthew. It will be very nice for just Susan and I to visit.

You can see Susan's pain when Matthew is visiting. Little things like holding him on her shoulder, burping him, walking with him to settle him down, are all not possible now, and may never be possible. Her present limitations are magnified with respect to taking care of Matthew.

I've said all along that we will figure out a way to do what we want and have Susan take care of Matthew as best as she can. Trying to do as much as she can and participating in his care as best as she can is all that we can do. To exaggerate the present limitations or to try and do something that is difficult, like dressing him, is not helpful. Do what you can and move on from there. Very easy to say. Extremely difficult to do.

This is the reality, but that doesn't make the reality any easier nor does it make Susan feel better about what she has missed and will likely miss doing with him. But the key is to be part of the process; a participant is best but an observer to events is better than nothing. Neither of us has to always be the doer, of course it is easy for me to say this since I can do everything with Matthew.

I have to switch to the mode of finding full-time help and all that it entails for home. Then there is the added responsibility of caring for Susan, but I need to remind myself that it's just "providing some help" on a temporary basis. Susan can do some things for herself and she just needs a little help with the rest. In time, she will be able to do more. That is the real value of time; it provides a mechanism for seeing possibilities which make one more hopeful.

All the insurance papers have been completed and filed. It will be interesting to see what happens with these claims. If all goes well, these claims will certainly help us financially until I no longer have to support Diane, my ex wife. There is also school for Amy and full-time help for us, so there is always going to be a drain on income. But we will get by, somehow we always do.

Things have quieted down in the house; Matthew fell asleep, Grandma is sleeping and Hans has been walked. I can have breakfast and read the paper or do some chores before I have to leave. One of the few moments each day when it is peaceful.

I'm hanging in pretty well. Doesn't sound like a strong endorsement, but it is the best I can do. I've not thought about it too much, but I've just done what had to be done. There hasn't been too much time to be reflective or to process feelings—you just do. I know at times I get very tired and just want to lie down or do nothing, but those moments pass. I'm sure Susan feels the same; she'd like this nightmare to be just that—a bad dream that is over and she can move on with her life. There are times when I think about what we wish could be versus what is. That distinction "what it was or could have been" versus "what is and might become" is an intellectual game that can either break you or make you. The less we focus on the past or what it could have been and confront the here and now while striving to make the future good and resolving/living with uncertainty, the better off we will be as individuals and as a couple. The past is only good if it helps you go forward. Every memory contains the joy of what we did, framed by the reality of what can be done now. This gap between memories and present reality is huge. Nevertheless, memories contain the joys of our lives and they are important to who we are – but they cannot become the measuring stick for who we will become.

When you feel sorry for yourself, you are remembering what it was or could have been. When you confront the situation and attempt to respond to it, you are acknowledging the present reality and going on from there. "Accept it" is not the correct phrase - acknowledge it; don't deny it; but certainly do not accept it. The task is to get on—move on with life. That's the challenge and task before us. It can only happen by meeting the daily challenges that present themselves. Getting on with our past life is impossible. Our life ended and we are trying to build a new one.

January 29 - Friday: 3:40 a.m.

Guess you could say that I'm up early! Matthew, after being on the war path during the night, finally fell asleep at 8:00 p.m. He was due for a bottle at 8:30, but I knew he'd never drink it when he was so tired.

Went to bed at 9:40 p.m. and he got up at 2:15 a.m. He was still in his clothes, so I had to change him and get him ready to eat. To make a long story short, he finally settled back down at 3:15 a.m. I walked the dog and here I am.

Doing his wash, making bottles, mailing some letters, and taking Hans for a walk. Lots of things to do and it's a quiet time. I know I'll pay for this later, but I'm awake now, so might as well do something.

A work-related meeting was scheduled downtown yesterday, but it was canceled. I decided to take my mom home and bring Matthew along for the ride to see Susan. Had a meeting with Institute of Psychiatry people about a project and I managed to convince a nurse to watch Matthew for awhile. It was a good chance to have a longer visit with Susan.

It's hard being a family when you can't be together to do things. We are approaching three months of being hospitalized and it is wearing thin. I'm beginning to wonder what is worse, the disability or the psychiatric toll it's having on Susan and me. It's not that she or I are nuts or anything, or that I'm loosing whatever mind I have left, it's just the institutionalization phenomena. When everyone who works at the hospital knows you at the hospital, it is too long. You've been there too long!

I surprised Susan about 10:00 a.m. She was finishing breakfast and was trying to get organized. Dr. Biller had a chance to see Matthew which was nice. We also looked at the CAT scan and the area of infection is about the same. This worries me. While it has reduced 30% from the original mass, it hasn't changed much since the last CAT scan. There is talk that the "wall" looks thinner (the shell of the encapsulated abscess), but this sounds like trying to find a silver lining. Susan is bothered by this report, as well. We just have to hope it will resolve, rather than dwell on what will or could happen if it does not.

I received the word that Susan is moving to rehab on Friday (today). A move anywhere (change of scenery) is great. This will help keep her going, although she wishes it was a move home—for good. Dr. Smith wants to see how she is doing and what catch-up work, if any, Susan has to do to get back to where she was and onward from there.

Matthew cooperated. He smiled as Susan fed him, plus all the doctors and nurses fussed over him. I know this makes her feel good, but the sad part is she feels she is not part of this or can't take credit for any of this. It's like she is just another visitor. I tried to tell Susan that without her, Matthew isn't here, so she has the biggest role of all to play.

With our "luck," Susan will be in the hospital for Matthew's three-month birthday, like she was for #1 and #2. If she is, I will surprise her with a cake or something to make it easier. I'll take Matthew downtown for his 3 month birthday party.

We spent a good part of the day downtown and I could tell she did not want us to leave, so we stayed until 2:00 p.m. Even at that, it was not enough because she is just devastated by not being home with us. It kills her to see us come and go so quickly. I try to put a smile on my face and joke about it, but I cry as Matthew and I walk back to the car. She doesn't know, but it's overwhelming for me to be home and not have her part of my life.

This second "brush with death" as Dr. Fernandez called it has taken its toll on Susan's confidence and belief that things will work out. I think she is now waiting for the "other shoe" or should I say **shoes** to drop. I'm not sure what the count is, but I told her that a fair number of shoes have already fallen. Her feeling is, "What's next?" There has to be something rather than this; it's over and we are on with living. Can't really say that I blame her. I have those thoughts as well. I mean, let's be real—things haven't gone well, so why should they start now. Simply put, they have to! We need a break, in order to have a chance. Susan needs time to regroup and get the feeling of joy for living and the desire to get her life back. We need this feeling—period. There has to be a sense of progress and hope just to get on with the struggle. It's hard to fight when you feel the fight is futile. Getting out of the hospital will be a huge boost to Susan's confidence. Once and for all she will be done with this place.

Harry Yates, the British wool representative who had a stroke and was at rehab during Susan's first go-round, called to see how she was doing. He sounded great. Things have worked out very well for him. He was shocked at Susan's setback. He called her and they had a good talk. I think it helped her confidence to see how far Harry had come.

Now that rehab is here, I have to think about what is next. Where can I find someone to help Susan and the baby? What kind of help does Susan need and want? Add to that the various ongoing trips and monitoring we are going to have to do over the next few months to keep us on the road to recovery. I need to find someone who is flexible, caring, and helpful – a saint.

I have an upcoming business trip, not exactly at the best time, as if there is any time now that is good. It's a chance to make about $1,000 which will help pay bills and whatever we might need.

I filed all the insurance papers. Geri, my secretary, did all the paperwork. Thank God for her help; the amount of paperwork is staggering.

Well I know I'll regret staying up later, but for now it has allowed me to catch up and get things done that need to be done.

January 30 - Saturday: 4:40 a.m.

Matthew had a bottle Friday night at 7:30 p.m. and slept until 3:00 a.m. He woke up, had a bottle, and is down again. But after being up 1½ hours, I'm up, so might as well write a bit. If I could get Matthew to take the last bottle at 10:00 p.m., then we'd be in business. Well that's one more thing to shoot for.

I am very busy at work. I barely have enough time to do anything other than meet and run. I had to take my expense forms to do over the weekend because I couldn't find the time to do them at work. I had to pick up my Mom at 1:30 p.m. and get back home, take her to her doctor's appointment and get back so Amy could use the car. Same story, run, run, run.

Susan moved to rehab! The abscess is still unchanged but according to Dr. Biller, Susan is making great progress. "Don't worry about the abscess," he said. "Work on walking and getting your strength back." The exact message Susan needed to hear. You are moving forward, making progress and you (Susan) are the reason for this improvement. Keep moving forward! Another step closer to coming home. Dr. Smith made the arrangements and Susan was fortunate to get placed in a two-bed room (things worked out). So, Susan is in the final home stretch of getting back on her feet (or foot), depending on one's level of cynicism.

If returning to the hospital was difficult, moving to rehab was more so. Rehab is not a fun place given all the broken lives you see. I am sure no one there ever thought they would be in such a place. We certainly didn't. I'm also sure everyone there wonders about what is going to happen to them; how will they deal with their injuries; and, when are they going to be able to leave. Clearly all the patients and their families face a life time of struggle and uncertain futures. The only thing that is certain is the life most had and knew is gone and won't be coming back. Such a collective sense of loss hangs over the place. People have stunned looks on their faces. All are thinking: "What will my life be like?"

The brain infection is still a problem. The abscess has reduced from its original size, but no noticeable changes since the last scan. I have a feeling this is an initial indication that another surgery is on the horizon. Even Dr. Smith said it's good Susan tolerates surgery well. Isn't that a great compliment! I wonder if they really think all these antibiotics will kill it or not? Dr. Biller does and he is convinced that if we hang in there long enough, it will resolve.

Susan needs a break. She does not need another surgery. I don't know how much more she can tolerate, let alone how likely she would become cognitively impaired as a result of the surgery. Two surgeries within three months on her head is two too many. Contemplating a third surgery is out of the question.

It must have been a zoo moving Susan—all her stuff, plus all the clothes and her wheelchair. Otto and Viola helped her. Her mother got bad news. It's clear Viola needs surgery on her neck, and the sooner the better. Not sure what she'll do, but it's just one more thing to think about. Viola has to have a surgical consultation and decide quickly. The longer Viola waits, the worse her overall condition will become. Plus, the ability to regain movement in her hands is maximized if the neck surgery is done now, rather than waiting.

Susan will come home on a pass today, but we really have to work around her twice-a-day antibiotics IV, which I will learn to do. Somehow, the antibiotic pod is hooked up to this central line in her chest for an hour in the morning and an hour in the evening for the next three weeks. This is serious, because of the importance of continuing treatment and the need to keep the line clear of infection. The central line has to be changed every week. An infection in the line, since it is near her heart, would be unthinkable.

The plan is to come home on the day I have to go to Florida. So now there is a real dilemma as to how to get Susan home, get help in the home for her and Matthew, plus get medical coverage for the IV line while I am away. One option is to have her stay a few extra days so that I will be returning home from the trip when she is coming home from Rehab. Not likely. I don't believe she would stay an extra moment let alone a day or so.

Talk about a logistical challenge. The added responsibility of her medical care scares me. I already feel like I have my hands full with Susan at rehab, Matthew, work and now I can add nurse to the list of things to do. I'm still trying to figure out whom to hire and, where to find them to help us when Susan gets home. How to pay them is a whole other matter. But, somehow it will work out and you can only do what you can do.

I'm worried about this lack of reduction in the brain infection. This uncertainty just adds high anxiety to the daily struggle.

Well, today is a great day. Susan can at least come home for awhile. It will be even better when it's for good and it will be the best when we know that we're on the way to full recovery. I'm confident that day will come.

February 2 - Tuesday: 6:25 p.m.

    I haven't written for a few days. Why even say no time, I should stop saying or writing that and get on with it.

    Susan was pumped Saturday. She could get out for at least a pass. After all this time, a pass sounded like a vacation. Out of the institution, back to familiar surroundings, sounds, smells, routines, normal people—a reality that's real, not like the institutional environment.

    As we left, we both started to cry. "I'm glad I'm alive and have all my marbles," Susan said. How true. Given other events, she could be worse off. There is a lady (almost brain dead) who had a heart attack, then a stroke during delivery. She is in Susan's old bed at rehab. It's hard to walk by and look at her without feeling her pain and, at the same time, be grateful for what we have. The baby survived and she has a 3-year-old at home in Indiana. I talked to her husband who indicated his wife was brain dead. He was waiting for family members to gather before removing life support. I can't imagine. I simply cannot imagine being in his situation.

    Susan enjoyed (what a bland word) being home; she was thrilled to be home and be with Matthew! She is surprised and in awe of the things he can do. She loves to watch him smile and he likes to do it for Mom.

    Being home is tiring. She does more walking and more transferring than she would at rehab. Plus, she is up and active, whereas she might catch a nap at rehab. It was a quiet day—we didn't do too much. Amy and Grandma went shopping and stopped by the house. Grandma cooked ribs for our early meal because Susan had to go back to rehab so that her antibiotic treatment could be given.

    Melinda and Susan's mom and dad also came by—they stayed for awhile and talked about all their respective ailments. Everyone sounded older than the next. I looked at Susan and said, "Who's nuts? Let's talk about health."

    Susan came home Sunday (Super Bowl Sunday) also. We shopped and bought some meat so we could cook a dinner Sunday afternoon. No one visited, in part, because Alisa has shingles, Amy went to a party, Joyce is out of town, and Betty has a cold. No one is really healthy. Susan is and prefers to stay that way.

Susan was vomiting in the morning at rehab and complained about a headache all day. She was told to take some Advil as needed. The headache worries her, as does the upcoming CAT scan. Hope the infection is reduced and reduced substantially. Susan doesn't want any other problems. She needs a break.

The good news is that February 5 is D-Day 2, the second discharge date. Everything has gone well at rehab and it's time to come home and restart our life. Susan will have home nursing care twice a day (a.m. and p.m.) for at least the next six weeks, along with physical/occupational therapy at home. The doctor indicated that insurance will cover home care and this is the best course of care for the next two to three weeks, until the antibiotics are done, the final CAT scan looks good and the IV comes out. That's the real date we are looking for, then (and with no further setbacks) we can get on with outpatient rehab and living.

She is ready! Susan would leave whether or not she was okayed to do so. Enough is enough and three-plus months of hospital life (except for the four days around New Year's) is enough. Like I said, she needs a break.

I have made arrangements for my out-of-town trip. Carole, her niece, will stay overnight and through Tuesday, until I return from Orlando. With luck, I will find someone to take care of Matthew and help Susan during the day. I have one lead and have discussed our needs with this woman. She'd like $60 per day or $300 per week. That's the going rate and there is little I (or anyone else) can do. We need help and there is nothing we can do or nothing that can be said to change this fact.

Susan and I hope to talk to this woman over the weekend and make a decision. There are not a whole lot of options available—this may work out. We'll have to see. I make this decision-making process sound more complicated than it really is. We either hire her or have no help. Not really a choice.

Work is okay. I'm worried about the company and whether or not the company can survive. There are some serious doubts about surviving, given what has been occurring in our line of work. Management at the health system is incensed at the leadership style of our "leader" —which is no leadership. Things are going to break apart real fast if the business can't be turned around.

I'm trying to line up new business and it is not easy with what is happening with Susan, the present workload, and the work that has to be done. Maybe the upcoming conference will give me a chance to explain the new business concept to a variety of potential customers.

I have to get Matthew up. I don't want him to sleep all evening and be up all night.

The Good News! Great News! On Friday, Round #2 starts. This time, there will be no setback. There is no turning back. We'll be looking and moving forward. Enough is enough. Home is where she is headed.

February 4 - Thursday: 6:40 p.m.

Not real good news. The CAT scan does not show any real reduction in the size of the abscess and Susan's white blood count is low. After the initial shrinkage, the abscess has remained unchanged. A low white count usually means an infection and even more ominous, the inability to fight the infection. Given all the antibiotics she has been receiving, an infection is the last thing she should have. No one seems to know why, but the bottom line is that she is not coming home as planned, and how long she'll have to stay in the hospital is unclear. The real underlying problem is this infection does not want to resolve itself and that may mean more surgery.

There are no words to explain this feeling of "will it ever end?"—"how much more can she take?"—"can she survive another surgery?"—"it's a nightmare!"—"what's next?" It goes on and on. Every time we attempt to plan ahead something happens and the plans change. There is no control in our life. Helpless and anxious characterize our feelings.

In talking with Susan tonight. I am positive and she is positive. There is no other way to be. As we talked, I told her now is not the time to "go south" (get depressed). She just has to keep fighting. She understands this and is extremely resilient. I know I would be over the edge by now. Susan isn't and that in itself is a miracle!

All the doctors have been wonderful. Dr. Biller even found Susan in her exercise class to tell her about the CAT scan. It had not reduced any appreciable amount. Why? Who knows? It just hasn't. But as he says, and says so confidently, "It will. It is like a prize fight where nothing is happening and the person is losing and all of a sudden in the 12th round he knocks out the opponent. We are in the 10th round. Still some time to go. It will resolve itself. Just have to wait it out." What a boost that was. Just what Susan and I, but especially Susan, needed to hear from someone with expertise – not just me. His remarks made staying in the hospital a whole lot easier.

Now with her white blood count low, she is susceptible to infections and may have to be placed in isolation, because her body cannot fight an infection. She doesn't need another problem like pneumonia or something worse.

I spent the day with her. I was able to take her to the CAT scan because my 11:00 a.m. appointment was canceled. Also, I wanted to pack up her belongings in anticipation of going home. Well, I did that and right now I'm washing her clothes so I can take them all back.

My guess is that we are looking at another week; ten days to make sure this white blood count is resolved. No sense having this continue to be a problem because it means she can't really fight infections anywhere.

Susan's initial reaction to this current medical problem was disbelief, disgust and a sense of being disheartened. Why not?! What else could/should it be? But I think she has turned the corner and knows where she stands and why she has to get this infection resolved. It's imperative! Information is vital to knowing where you stand and what you are willing to do. Not staying or attempting to leave early would be a set back to her. She understands that. Susan simply doesn't like the way staying feels.

Grandma will watch Matthew at her place on Monday while I'm out of town. I can't believe I have to leave, but I need to make the outside money, so there is really no choice. I will be gone just overnight, so it will not be that long. I will get Matthew when I return.

Matthew is going to go to Betty's on Friday night and Joyce's on Saturday night so I can get some sleep and be downtown more. Matthew being cared for will be helpful and allow me to be downtown with Susan to give her support over the weekend.

Not much more to say. This is a real setback, but one that can be overcome. As an aside, Susan has made real strides in her walking and use of her arm. She now can bend her ankle which she couldn't before. The ankle goes down but Susan cannot make it come up. This is something she could not do before. In time she may regain the full range of the ankle/foot movement. She has made great progress and this infection is not going to stop her!

February 7 - Saturday: 8:10 p.m.

When you think things can't get any worse, well they can! No breaks have come our way. That's not to say we aren't grateful. Susan is alive and has her marbles; but we need a break to get on with our life.

Not only did Susan not come home, she didn't have a weekend pass. "I can't really go home with that low white blood count," she said. "Too many germs at home." But, I thought, isn't there a host of germs in the hospital? Not going home for a visit is almost unbearable. She is close to breaking (giving in), as it gets harder and harder to stay away from home. She knows it and so do I.

Matthew being at Betty's and then Joyce's allowed me to get some things done that I've been unable to do, like buying shoes and going to the cleaners, doing some shopping and picking up Matthew's pictures. These are the pictures taken at Sear's on the day of the big snow. They turned out very well. These are his three-month-old birthday pictures. I hope Susan likes them.

Once I got things organized, I went downtown and spent the day with Susan. It was nice to be alone and talk, as well as not talk, but be together. Didn't do anything special. Susan couldn't leave the building. We shared a hamburger, popcorn, and mint chocolate-chip ice cream. One of our better balanced meals.

Susan and I had a sort of review of life talk. Where are we at? Where are we going? The future of so many things is uncertain: her ability to regain independence, caring for Matthew, the fear of more surgery, the infection and its inability to resolve itself. Small talk! Nothing but minor issues.

When she started to talk about her hand and how she hoped she could do things like take care of Matthew and bake cookies for him, I broke down. I don't really think I have cried in front of her before, but I was just so overwhelmed by her courage and the struggle she is in that I just broke down. It took awhile for me to compose myself.

At another point, we were talking and I asked if she had to go to the bathroom. I'd never think of asking her that in my wildest dreams—but now I do. I told her I had to stop doing that. I apologized—she is a big girl. She knows if she needs to go or not. Why do I ask? So I told her she can ask me if I have to go the bathroom if that would make her feel any better. She said she would and she would also ask me if I washed my hands.

We talked about this change in roles and identified an interesting process. She is independent and dislikes being unable to do things her way. I don't want to wait for her to ask for things all the time, so I naturally will say, "want a coke?" or "Kleenex?" or whatever. This makes it easy for her, since she is not always having to ask. So it's natural to add bathroom.

She broke down when she said that she knew she wasn't the "woman I married." "Not so," I stated. This is only true in a slight physical sense. More than ever, she is the woman I married! The things I love about her are what she still has. Her laugh, her wit, her mannerisms. Just the way we get along. That's who I married, that's who she is and why I love her. So nothing—nothing has changed. There are obstacles to overcome, but we can confront them as they happen.

The medical team is still trying to figure out the infection. Susan was extremely disappointed that she couldn't leave on a pass today. But the white blood cell count is low and getting lower. That scares her, plus the possibility of more surgery. If this abscess can't be resolved through antibiotics then surgery is the only option left.

While Matthew and Hans are sleeping, I'll sit in silence for awhile. It's nice to have some quiet.

February 8 - Monday: 3:30 p.m.

I'm at O'Hare and ready to fly to Orlando. First trip since the baby. Lots of things to organize to get ready to go. Matthew is at Grandma's in the city; Hans is being cared for by Amy (she has the car); Susan is downtown; so everything seems to be set.

Susan called this morning and said she might be leaving Tuesday. I went into a rage, since it's another thing to organize and coordinate. I'm at the point of feeling overwhelmed and there is so much to do and only me to do it. To learn she may be leaving the hospital while I am boarding the plane put me over the edge.

I know I was yelling at Susan. I apologized, but I had about had it. I mean, she couldn't come home Sunday because of her low blood count and at 8:00 a.m., on Monday, Dr. Smith says she might go home Tuesday. Susan didn't even have the lab values. How could she go home if she couldn't have a weekend pass? Then there is all the home care to arrange, plus the sitter to take care of her and Matthew. That lady is to start next Monday, not this Wednesday. There has to be better planning for all of this to happen. I cannot be told in the morning that everything changes after making the plans based on another set of circumstances, and now I am about to board a flight.

Matthew was fed at 10:30 p.m. last night; got up at 2:00 a.m.; then got up at 5:30 a.m. and remained up. He is spitting up the formula too much. I called the pediatrician and he was switched to soybean. Grandma got a couple of cans and I exchanged all the Enfamilᶢ cans for Prosoybee. Have to see how that works. Now as a satisfied kid, he'll feel better without all the gas pains he has had.

Matthew seems to spit up constantly (maybe quite a bit is less of an exaggeration), plus he won't give up screaming. He stops

163

if I come by and/or he sees me and is picked up. I put him down and he goes nuts. Gas or not, it is impossible to do wash, pack, pack him up, clean up, start laundry, walk Hans, pack myself/himself, do dishes, and talk on the phone. I do feel overwhelmed. You would think I would realize this by now and being overwhelmed would be second nature, normal, but as tasks mount I feel the weight. You would also think that by now I would realize the nature of the situation and just go with the flow. The phrase "can't teach an old dog new tricks" seems appropriate.

Somehow I have to lighten up—not get uptight. This is easier said than done. Maybe swimming or some type of exercise will help. I have to do something to relieve this pressure/tension. I can't imagine why I ever said swimming. I can't swim. Maybe this is a secret death wish – like I would drown if I ever took up swimming.

Susan sounded better today. At least it is busy and there are things to do compared to the weekend. Weekends are a death sentence at the rehab center—without visitors and therapy appointments, time stands still. Yesterday, Susan found herself at breakfast with three seniors at least twice her age and wrestling being shown on the TV. Nobody wanted wrestling, but it was noisy and movement to watch and the cleaning staff were into wrestling. All the rooms have the same channel on so that wrestling can be enjoyed by the few who want to watch it. Even though you may want quiet or something else on the TV, you can't do or say anything about it. Voice an opinion and you quickly find out why it is the last time you do that.

Susan said she got depressed when she said to herself that she hoped she wouldn't be like them, her 80-year-old tablemates. Yet, here she is at 38, and in many ways like them. No wonder why she worries about what the future will bring. Anybody with their right mind would worry about this. It's real and no one has any answers. That's what's scary. She has rightly noted that even with half her brain gone she is keenly aware of what worst-case possibilities exist.

I will probably take a couple of days off until Monday when Maria, the caregiver hired to help us, arrives. That should give us time to establish a routine and food and stuff into the house.

I talked with Susan again before I left Chicago and she is not as optimistic about leaving on Tuesday. Why get your hopes up when, at the last minute, they change the plans. We truly should take things a day at a time, there is no choice—that's just how things are. You take things a day at a time because there is no option to do otherwise; maybe that's too big of a time span.

Well the plane is ready to board, so I'll stop for awhile. I'll call Susan when I get to Orlando.

February 10 - Wednesday: 9:00 p.m.

Well things can't get worse. Like I said before, when you think it can't, it does.

I got a migraine headache flying back from Florida, so I was really out of it and went to the ER, along with Matthew who had been throwing up when he was at Grandma's and my sister, Betty's. I didn't get home until 1:00 a.m.

What a homecoming for Susan. Of course, Susan arrived to this "zoo." I arrived home before she did and was able to put her sign up: "Welcome Home Susan! Again!" So at least she got to see it. But as soon as she arrived, she could tell I wasn't right. She has seen my "migraine look" before. There is nothing I can do to stop it once it starts. The only thing that works is to vomit and try to sleep. But I couldn't sleep, given all the commotion going on. The home nurse stopped by, her mother and dad were here and I was out of it.

The home nurse took my blood pressure and it was higher than a kite (160/98). All I need is a stroke. Susan was out of her mind with fear over Matthew and me. So off to the ER he and I went.

Chapter 7
HOME AGAIN

"Faithless is he who says farewell when the road
darkens."

- J R Tolkin

February 12 – Friday: 5:35 a.m.

After 3½ months, Susan comes home to chaos. I was useless. I knew the migraine was starting on the plane and there was nothing I could do about it. I tried aspirin, but once it gets going, forget it.

I tried to sleep, vomit, and/or bury my head, but nothing worked. Only time, sleep and enough vomiting does the trick. Eventually, I went to the ER with Matthew. Betty and John took us. Never was seen by a physician in the ER due to the rush of work, so I fell asleep; woke up and felt better. We (Matthew and I) left the ER and got home at 1:00 a.m. and went to bed.

Joyce, Chris (Susan's sister-in-law and brother) and Viola were at the house when I arrived from the ER. Susan tried to stay up, but couldn't. I think she was glad we (Matthew and I) were home and okay.

I feel exhausted. I have been running and doing whatever has to be done. I really have to decide what to do about this migraine problem because I can't let it get out of control, or worse, blow a blood vessel.

Both Wednesday and Thursday, Susan, Matthew, and I did a lot of running around. I didn't go to work either day. I took Matthew to the pediatrician. He is fine and gaining weight. Betty and John took care of him on Tuesday night. There are a lot of things to do with the home nurse and OT. Someone is always coming and going. This is the best set-up. Let Susan receive her antibiotic care at home until the infection is resolved and the central line can be removed.

It is sort of ironic that the driving force that kept Susan going and working hard was to get home to be Matthew's Mom. However, arriving at home proved to be very depressing for her. Home made Susan's limitations crystal clear. The hope of being home, taking care of him, doing things, clashes with the reality of the home experience itself.

The home Susan left over three months ago is not the same because she is not the same. What was done before can't be done now. Experiencing this reality produces a sense of profound sadness and loss.

Susan is confined to a wheelchair, except for very simple transfers to the toilet and bed. Carpeting prevents her from trying to be mobile in the wheelchair. Pulling herself with her right foot and pushing with her right hand places a strain on these limbs and gives an imbalance to the chair at times. The chair looks as if it is going around in a circle.

Susan is trying to participate in taking care of Matthew. While "participate" may seem like an awkward word to describe her activities, it is reflective of what she is able to do at this time. Susan tries to establish the schedule, identify things to do, and as much as possible tries to participate in accomplishing these tasks, especially where Matthew is involved. Whatever she can do she does and then some.

Susan is doing real well, but is very tired and exhausted from all that has happened. Keep in mind she still has a significant brain infection. She is trying to get her rest without worrying too much about what's going on in her head. What will happen if that abscess doesn't resolve itself is anybody's guess. I just can't see more surgery; that would put all of us over the edge. I know this sounds like a broken record, but it is the only "music" playing in our heads. All the time.

Susan went for a CAT scan on Thursday. We don't know anything yet. I will try and find out the results. I dropped Matthew off at Grandma's, which made everything a bit easier.

It is a busy day around the house with the nurses, Matthew, Hans and what has to get done, but all-in-all things are going well. We have to figure out some type of schedule to the chaos in order to get everything done that needs to be done.

I'm going to work today. Dora and Amy are coming to be with Susan. That should give everyone some help until I get home in the early evening. Work is a series of decisions all aimed at keeping us employed. Also, all the insurance papers have to be re-filed. Once is not good enough. I assume the reason for the refilling requests is to see if the person is serious. Sort of a test. Never before have I experienced the insanity of "claims." The only thing I have learned is that the insurance companies try to "claim you have no claim." If the claim is rejected ten times these insurance companies hope you just give up.

I felt sad when I was in Orlando just seeing families walking around and running after their kids. Are we really going to be able to do this? Will Susan be able to? Right now it kills her not to be able to take care of Matthew. Little things like holding him, walking with him, patting his back. The basics of caring for him are not doable by her now. To see her struggle with that is quite painful. The more she tries, the more she realizes what she cannot do. But that doesn't stop her from trying, so give her credit. She is not a quitter. I don't think she knows the meaning of the word.

Maria, the lady who will help us, starts Monday. We will have to see how that works out. I'm sure it will be an adjustment. I just hope it works so we can get some kind of regular help at home, which we desperately need. I expressed a hope that this person will work out, knowing it will be difficult for her to "help but not take over," "ask rather than decide," etc. Finding someone to help a person live her life rather than to control her life is a challenge. Very few people would choose to "live with help," so that should tell you how difficult this is.

February 14 - Sunday: 5:05 a.m. - Valentine's Day

Things keep moving forward, but there was no good news about the CAT scan. The abscess is the same size as when the antibiotics were started. There has been no reduction past the initial change. This makes surgery a real possibility. Hard to believe this is the only option. Plus, how many times can you have brain surgery without causing more trouble?

There are plenty of ups and downs. We went shopping at a local mega-mall on Saturday, but it is not the same. First, I'd never go shopping. Second, Susan is independent and would go and do as she pleased, but the chair really prevents that. So here we are, doing things we don't enjoy. But, as I told Susan, "at least we are sharing the misery together."

It is not that easy to get around with the crowds and aisles and the stairs as they are, but it wasn't too bad either. Just bittersweet. Susan struggles with her dependence on others versus her independent streak. When she was putting her makeup on this morning, the baby started crying and I was in the process of taking the dog out. She said, "I just sat and waited till you were done. I could not do anything to comfort him. So I sat and cried along with him until you came back to us."

Trapped—that's how we all feel—that's what we are. She needs help and Matthew and I need help. I can't do anything unless I figure out who could watch them and stay with them if I went to the store or did some errands. So we are all in the same boat, we just have different views, but at least we are in the same boat together!

We have talked about being overwhelmed by our feelings. What can we do to feel better? These feelings of loss, sadness, helplessness, dependence, uncertainty, and add any word I might have missed, are a weight on our minds. They are always present. How heavy they feel varies by the moment and the event. It is not really easy or clear for anybody. Add to this Susan's inability to do a whole lot for Matthew. Feeding is about it—very frustrating. Just the same, it is a beginning.

Today we are having a birthday party for Melinda, as well as a little Valentine's Day celebration. I've ordered all the food, so it won't be that big of a deal—at least I hope not.

Never any time, always far more to do, or help to give, or whatever, than there is the ability to give it. Cleaning, washing, the baby, cooking, etc., is more than a full-time job. With this lady starting, it should make things easier; at least that is my hope. I have a full week at work, so we will see how this goes.

I'll call the doctors on Monday to see what the follow-up plans are. Susan has a Friday appointment for another CAT scan and an evaluation. She stops her antibiotics on Thursday and then we will find out what the next course of action is.

Susan just needs good news. Some type of good news to get her over the hump. She can't face the prospect of another surgery. Surgery right now is impossible. Who am I kidding? Any surgery is impossible whether it is now or later.

February 17 - Wednesday: 6:25 p.m.

Time to get back to what's been happening. Maria, the lady who is helping us, started Monday (2/15/93). I had hired her when Susan was still hospitalized and hoped she'd work out. Susan and I never were able to see her (interview her) or talk with her about our expectations, so Maria started sight unseen. After three days, I think she has worked out ok, not sure this sentiment is shared by Susan. I'm not sure Mother Teresa would work out in such a situation. Her retort was pure Susan: "Living with one saint is hard enough; I don't think I could handle two."

Maria is very eager to work, keeps busy and takes care of Matthew. She is very caring and affectionate toward him which makes a bad situation almost tolerable for Susan. Notice I said "almost tolerable." Maria likes Matthew, but her caring for Matthew is heartbreaking for Susan. It is a constant source of pain for Susan to see someone care for and love her child in a way that she can never do - pick him up when he's hurt, walk with him to calm him down—it is the ultimate cruelty. But love and caring can be demonstrated and felt in different ways. In an odd sort of way, the better Maria is with Matthew, the worse it is for Susan. His needs are now. Needs change and Susan will have lost an ability to care for him at this unique age. As he grows, though, there will be other opportunities. I am confident that Susan will find a way to connect, to feel like his Mom by doing things only Moms can do.

Susan was upset Monday when Maria arrived because it clearly meant she needed help and someone else (instead of her) was going to take care of Matthew. Not her! And, that's her problem. She can't do these things – for Matthew and the home when I am at work. So someone had to be hired. It doesn't make it any more tolerable. But to be actually confronted by this reality – a stranger who is paid to help Susan and take care of Matthew is a shock. Susan's realization that she needs help, help from anyone, let along Maria is difficult to accept, like, or want. The reality of a paid caregiver only adds insult to injury. Who among us would like to be in this situation?

Practically everything that Matthew needs or Susan would like to do with him can't be done by her. While that is painful enough, to see others (including myself) do these activities and play with him, simply adds to the pain. She is the outsider in her role as a mother and not really the mom she had planned to be. If this doesn't break her heart, nothing will – ever! I have to find ways for her to feel more in control of what happens with Matthew. She has to feel like his mom and everyone has to recognize that Susan is Matthew's mom.

Trying to juggle work, home, and everything in-between is a trick. Maria helps by doing a lot of what has to be done. Matthew is cooperating and sleeps from 9:00 or 10:00 at night until 5:00 or 5:30 in the morning. Very, very good for him.

Money has become a real issue. I called the bank on Monday and learned we had $47 total – in checking, two bucks short of my age. That is the total sum of our funds. No savings or a Christmas Club account. Just $47 period. I received an expense check that will be somewhat helpful. Any source of money from anywhere is welcomed.

Susan and I are getting into a routine. It's been hard to figure out who should do what and when. It is not easy to decide the new subtleties of a relationship. For example, should I always ask if she wants anything or should I wait for her to ask? Do I wait outside the bathroom so she doesn't have to call me or do I give her more privacy and wait for her to call, hoping that I hear her? The examples are endless. There are no rules. You make them up as you go. You change them often. There are no rules.

February 18 - Thursday: 5:07 a.m.

Matthew got up at 3:30 a.m., in part because he was up all day and went down for a nap at 7:00 p.m. last night. In any event, he was up early and I stayed up. Lots of little things to catch up on, like this diary.

I have been trying to get the insurance/disability forms completed and re-filed. Nothing is simple with these people. If every "i" and "t" is not dotted or crossed, everything stops dead in its tracks. Forms have to be submitted at least three or four times. I often feel this is a contest to see who will say "uncle" first.

Geri, my secretary, has been real helpful in completing all the forms so all the paperwork has been taken over by her. Thank goodness for the help. These forms come in daily and it's almost a full-time job keeping up with things.

I have had to talk to the lawyer about Dr. Toig's inability and/or unwillingness to help provide copies of records so that disability insurance claim forms can be completed. I hope to gain his cooperation and get on with filing claims.

I am trying to coordinate Susan's antibiotic care. There is a little confusion as to who is in charge. Dr. Biller wants to extend the home care beyond today—until at least we see what's going on with the infection and what can be done next. It makes sense to me, but not to the insurance company. Insurance has told me this "event" is costing a lot of money. Can you imagine? This "event" is costing a multi-billion dollar company a lot of money. They should ask my wife what the "event" has cost.

Friday, we are going to see Dr. Biller. The big question is what to do? What's next, given the abscess and what has already been tried? Susan does not want to run the risk of additional seizures, nor do we want any more surgery. Twice is enough. Susan has seen what can happen and go wrong; she doesn't want to take any more chances. While her "luck" is not exactly good, she is all together and with it. Her fear, besides death (can you imagine having death as a real possibility, and thus a fear?) is that some cognitive impairment and/or permanent paralysis beyond what she is dealing with is a distinct possibility with any additional surgery. These "results" don't make us eager to rush into surgery. She is an informed consumer of health care. I think she probably would qualify for an honorary MD degree. Our hope is no more surgery and with time the abscess will resolve.

Thoughts of going through all this a third time blow me away. I know, or should I say, I can imagine what Susan thinks about, if I have these feelings of "you've got to be kidding," what must she think?

I have a meeting downtown today. Could be new business. I have to find ways of getting new business.

Matthew is up with me now and he is so tired. He had gone back to bed after his 3:30 a.m. bottle. Well, I think he is up for awhile. Sounds like he is shitting in his bouncer chair, while I write. At least he is regular.

February 21 - Sunday: 5:45 a.m.

Friends, who we haven't seen since Matthew was born, are coming by for a visit today. It snowed quite a bit so we'll have to see what happens. They may not wish to make the trip to our home in the snow.

Susan had the CAT scan Friday and it is basically unchanged. Less swelling, but the infection/abscess still is unresolved. She is going to try another two weeks of IV antibiotics and hope for the best. On March 5, Susan will have another CAT scan and will have the central line taken out. Who knows what will happen; we'll just have to wait it out.

Friday was a long day. We left at 9:00 a.m. and got home at 4:30 p.m. CAT scan broke down and Susan had to wait two hours on the table. Doctors were late because they wanted to see the pictures and had to walk back from their offices to take a look.

I got checked out for migraines and that's about what they are. I was given some medicine to take at their onset. I hope that helps.

We tried to have lunch with Renee (Susan's primary nurse at rehab), but that didn't work given the time bind we were in. We will try again. Nurses and therapists are still coming for home care throughout the day (and night for that matter); always a large group in our home.

The doctors sound confident. We don't have a choice. It's either the antibiotics or and we're not sure what the "or" is or when the "or" can occur. I think it will be a conservative course of action. Susan will complete the course of antibiotic treatments and then wait it out.

Things have been going great at home. Susan is doing extremely well walking. She does a lot better (her form, speed, pointing toes, etc.) without the cane than with it. I don't know why that's the case, but it is. Also, her hand is not as tight and there is no need for the brace to be put on the hand at night.

Like I said, everybody comes and goes. My mother, her friend, the nurse, Betty and John, neighbors, physical and occupational therapists and the nurse again, all were over on Saturday; a slow day when you think Maria is not even here.

We are still adjusting to how to do things and how to get everything done that needs to get done. At times, I lose my patience and ability to just take things as they come. Last night at dinner, I was cooking, Matthew was yelling, and Hans wanted to eat - all at the same time. I then lost patience with Matthew which made Susan upset.

We talked about how overwhelming this is. I have to do most, if not all, of everything now and at times I reach my limit. But I have to state this and not feel guilty about saying, "I've had it." If Susan just says, "Okay Bill, just slow down," that's the clue for me to realize that things are starting to get out of hand. At that point, I need to step back and go with a time out. Otherwise, it will drive me nuts—and her.

We all know insight is a wonderful thing and talk is cheap. Will have to see how events play out. I have to be better able at just letting things go, take a breather/count to 10 and start over.

With all that was going on, I didn't even clean up because there was another thing to do or something to get organized. Plus, I just can't do things when I want to. Matthew and Susan can't be left alone so someone has to stay if I go out or Matthew comes with while Susan stays at home. So you wait around a lot for help and then try and get as much done as you can.

When we were downtown for the CAT scan, we ran into a lot of people we knew (transporters, nurses, residents, etc.). It's like they have seen us so much, we belong.

February 23 - Fat Tuesday: 6:20 a.m.

I'm real tired, plus my back is sore. While shoveling snow, I must have pulled some muscles. No big deal, but that's the most physical work I've done in three-plus months. I need to figure out how to exercise—try and get back in shape.

Last night I was very tired. A host of responsibilities. Since this nightmare won't end, I have to figure out how best to do what has to be done. Sometimes I wake up and think "well, I'll go to the 'Y' and Susan will probably do" Then I remember the reality that nobody is going anywhere and Susan can't do as much as she would like to – at least not yet. Sleep gives us a break from the press of the daily experiences.

It wears on you, day-in and day-out—I can only imagine what it is like for Susan. Wondering how each day will go and if she'll get back more functionality. What will the day and next week hold? What about the abscess? What about the future? The bills, you name it and the questions go on and on. There is no relief from the "what about" or "will I" questions. Just have to realize these questions are unanswerable. Living without structure, control, and answers is difficult. This is truly limbo, it only increases one's anxiety and fears about tomorrow.

I'm glad Maria has turned out well so far (notice I say so far because one never knows). Doubt if Susan sees this the same way I'm waiting for something to happen, because it has just been too good to be true. No matter how good the situation is or appears to be, how good can it be to have someone help you do things you use to do before, or care for your son? Notice, this is my perspective. I am not sure Susan would share the same sentiment about how well things are going. Let's just say they are going.

Work is a pain in the ass. The company is failing and I'm trying to figure out how to survive. Not real interested in devoting effort to work. The lack of security and job stability is just insane. Yet, you are powerless to do anything, because you can't do what has to be done.

By the end of the day, that typically starts at 4:00 a.m., I have lost whatever humor I had. That's when Matthew starts his fussy time, of course. Why would it be any other way? He is really very good; aside from his gas he is a happy, good-natured baby. Susan is doing more with him and for him, but it still is very hard for her. The gap between what she wants and would like to do, and can do, is enormous. Her struggle to live with this gap each

177

day is painful to watch. As Matthew gets older, this gap will widen because she may not be able to run after him, pick him up, and do all the things she wants to do. We both know that each stage of his development through life will present its own set of unique problems. Susan is up to the challenge of meeting them head-on.

Matthew (babies in general) are a lot of work (I have forgotten how much work). At times, I just want a break and not to have to do anything for anyone, not even myself. I even resent Hans, our dog, wanting a treat or water every time I have four or five other things to do. It's this constant demand and total responsibility that is just too much. Try as I might to just roll with what can or can't be done, what doesn't get done is waiting to be done sooner or later. When someone says, just let it go, my question is—till when?

Things will probably settle down once all the nursing stuff ends in another ten days or so. Then we wait and see what will happen to the abscess and what options are available to resolve it. For all I know, Susan can live with it so long as it does not affect her health or daily activities.

As I sat writing, I fell asleep. I'm sure I could sleep on command. But it's time to shovel the snow. We had a nine inch storm last night. Just when we thought winter was over, it came again with its full fury. Sort of like early January in late February.

Maria is coming in late because I have to stay late tonight for management meetings.

March 5 - Friday: 6:05 a.m.

It's been a long time since I've had a chance or the time to make any notes in the diary. Time is something I don't have. I've said it before, but it's true, there is simply no time to do all that <u>has</u> to be done, let alone have time to do anything you'd want or like to do. I'm not talking a round of golf or anything. I mean go for a walk or run with the dog. Even Hans can't go for his walks and he barely gets outside to shit.

Today is CAT scan day; Doctor Day; stop the treatment and wait day. The eight-week course of antibiotics stops today and the central line comes out—what's next is anybody's guess. We just hope the abscess or whatever it is will have resolved itself. Time will tell, so we have to wait. Time is something we have in this situation.

Susan is making progress. Earlier in the day she was exhausted, because I think she overdid it. Too much walking, multiple physician appointments, and staying up late. She had a tough time walking—a setback in her steady progress. But that has come around and things seem okay. She still has a shoulder that is killing her. With luck, it won't get any worse and she can get back to her exercises.

Matthew continues to grow. He laughs a lot and is a very happy baby. Always smiling, laughing and enjoying life. His gas problems have lessened, which just contributes to his overall good mood – perhaps to mine as well.

Susan has far more good days than bad moments, but every day there are the reminders. She can't hold him, dress him, or walk with him. She can help with all of these, but it is not the same or what she planned on doing.

She talks about giving away her shoes and clothes, like she will never wear these clothes again. I'm joking with her, but symbolically she is trying to get the home in order before she dies. From her point of view, I'm sure there are times (probably more times than I'd care to know about) when she feels like she has already died. Some days she goes through the motions and that is very wearing on her. Given the orthopedic device on her left foot, she will never wear any of her high-heeled shoes again. I am not sure about the clothes. But, as only Susan would point out, "A dress suit with white clown gym-shoes has yet to become a fashion craze."

Susan had her hair and nails done. She doesn't like the hairstyle, but there is nothing she can do about it. The hair has to grow and there isn't enough of it to work it into a decent hair style. So she looks like that Irish singer, Sinead O'Connor. It is a look she can pull off.

Susan is homebound and refers to any trip outside of the house, regardless of the time and/or destination, as an outing. She doesn't go anywhere any more. Clearly not by herself, so she has taken to referring to these activities as outings or field trips. Just like at rehab, patients went out every once in awhile. The same is true for Susan at home. As you might expect, she is unhappy with this state of affairs. What she has been wanting is an outing.

The routine around the house is set. Everything depends on Matthew cooperating, but by and large, we cook, eat, clean up and shower with little trouble. It takes time and organization, but with practice, we have figured out how to do almost everything that we want or need to do with as little or as much help as we need!

The flow of traffic has been non-stop: nurses in the a.m. and p.m.; OT/PT every other day; Maria, family/friends; delivery of health care products. It's almost around the clock. The experience with the nurses has been real good. It has worked out very well; they are pleasant and professional.

Maria still continues to be acceptable. She has taken on a great deal of the household work and that has given me a break. She also has been extremely sensitive and helpful to Susan and in the care she gives to Matthew. It couldn't have turned out any better, again, at least at this point in time. Things may change and I'm sure they will. Keep in mind this is me talking and not Susan. I'm sure Susan has a different perspective on Maria.

There are things to do before Matthew gets up and Maria arrives. I will report later about the doctor visits and the plan.

March 10 - Wednesday: 5:15 a.m.

"The abscess is significantly reduced and there is a marked decrease in size." That's what Dr. Biller said last Friday. The words we have been living to hear!

Now you'd think we'd be thrilled—and we are—<u>but</u> the real question that popped up immediately is "will it stay that way when the medications are withdrawn?" It's almost like good news is hard to take or not tolerated very well since there always seems to be another shoe about to drop.

I don't know what we expected to hear last Friday. We didn't want to talk about another surgery or even think about it. Maybe we knew or felt the abscess would resolve, I don't know. The real issue since the medication has stopped, will be in one month (April 2); when we learn whether the abscess is gone for good or growing again.

Susan has been Betty BoBo lately; my name for her when she feels depressed. More and more, she realizes her limitations and her inability to do things for herself and Matthew. Coming to terms with that is difficult, since it hits you in the face every day. There is no break from this reality. Every action reminds you of what can't be done, what has to either be relearned or done differently – or done for you by someone else.

Melinda was over and Susan feels/knows that things are different with her best friend. They can't do the things they did; she doesn't feel like her old self with Melinda. Therein lays the bind. Susan and I talked a great deal about what to do: 1) hope she will return to normal; or 2) realize this is it, it won't get better. What? Regardless of which option, or combination of options she chooses, she still moves forward. Depression is what it is. Nevertheless, Matthew is a great motivator since she wants to do as much as she can for him.

She acknowledges that she will <u>never</u> be the same. She emphasizes <u>never</u>! But do you dwell on that or use the past as a benchmark? In reality, what other benchmark do you have except that record of who you were and what you did? On the other hand, a new ball game is being played. There are new rules, expectations, and goals. So what do you do? You either play or sit down. Susan is a player!

Add to these issues of uncertainty about health, threat of surgery, and hope that is tested daily, the fact that she has shoulder and hip problems just adds to the mess. Her separated shoulder (caused by a fall during physical therapy) has prevented her from doing some of the things she'd like to do, as well as the hamstring (the result of using her one good leg to dig into the floor to propel the wheelchair forward). So now she has these nagging physical problems, in addition to the rest. Physical problems are always going to be a concern since there is so much wear and tear on her remaining right leg, arm, and hand. I am sure she has thought of the unthinkable—losing the use of her right hand would leave her with no hands! I have, so I know she certainly must have.

181

Viola, Susan's Mother, has been scheduled twice and canceled twice for neck surgery. She has a bladder infection that has persisted. They will do more tests to see what is happening, and perhaps next week the operation can be scheduled. Of course, that's when Chris (Susan's brother) and I are out of town.

Matthew is as happy as can be, has more of a personality, and his hair is coming in so it looks like he has a crew cut. He is very good—very little trouble. He had been sleeping until 5:00 or 5:30 a.m., except for the past two days when he has been up at 3:30 or 4:00 a.m.

Work continues to be work. I'm trying to find a way to get on top of things; I will talk to the higher-ups in the company to see what is possible. I would like someone to see the value in separating us from the other elements of the company and allowing us to be a small research company.

We're looking for a car; hope to get a Taurus wagon. We'll see if all the paperwork and double-checking of credit allows us to get the car. We have our fingers crossed. We need a wagon for all our stuff (buggy, wheelchair, diaper bag, etc.) and Amy would just love to have our car to do whatever she has to do.

Susan is getting house crazy. While in the hospital, she said she would be so glad to get home. Well now that she is home, she sits in the wheelchair at the kitchen table (that's about the extent of it). She just has to get out more and do shopping/walking when the weather is nice. Home can be a prison just like anywhere else. It's not like she doesn't want to go out. Her health and the actual process of getting organized to go anywhere are challenging.

Family life is in flux. This is a nice way of saying we don't know who can do what first. Most days you go through the motions because you can't believe it—or there is so much to do that it is just overwhelming. Yet, you move forward. What else can you do? If you stop, you'll get run over for sure. So the motto is keep moving forward. If you stop, you'll become a target.

I am still dealing with the medical insurance, disability insurance, Social Security, lawyers and the hospital to obtain Susan's medical records. Why does it have to be so difficult to obtain a copy of her record?

March 16 - Tuesday: 6:15 a.m.

I've been up since 4:00 a.m. I'm not sleeping well, but the lack of sleep doesn't really bother me until late evening.

Regardless, I'm up, Matthew is sitting with me and there are a few free moments—these are rare. He sits in his bouncer on the table and watches me write. I occasionally make a noise or something and he will look away from the toys hanging above his head. Also, I am careful. I know he is on the table but he is not going to bounce anywhere.

Susan has an appointment to see Dr. Smith today. Her shoulder is killing her and even to me it looks bad. The arm hangs and the upper arm bone is pulling away from the shoulder. I know she is frustrated and is in a lot of pain; I hope she can get some relief.

Susan hasn't been real happy lately; not that she should be ecstatic or overjoyed. But there is a sense of futility, resignation and fatalism to her that casts a definite depressive tone. We try and talk about it. "Why talk?" Susan will often ask. Not a real receptive response.

I can't blame her. On the other hand, what are we going to do about it? She is very tired and a big part of her tiredness are the drugs she takes. Also, these drugs affect her mood state. These feelings of "what is the use?" will not go away and it is something we have to confront as best we can. I have similar feelings myself. Perhaps we can learn from each other.

As the days pass, there is less enthusiasm about her ultimate progress. She has this six-month window in her head. If things will come back, they will do so in six months. Well, she takes that to be the ultimate truth. The abscess has been a setback, plus Susan has felt all along she'd be ahead of where she presently is if this abscess had not occurred. So, from her perspective, she is behind where she would have been if the abscess did not occur. And she is losing ground each day.

Losing ground each day is an interesting idea, since we weren't too sure what the future would hold. How does one know if one is ahead or behind? It is puzzling. The standard is always what you were and would/could have become. Now robbed of that dream, as well as that benchmark, she struggles with the uncertainty of what gauge to use in measuring progress. Always believing it will be better, but really not knowing if it will, and actually experiencing that it isn't much better. In spite of the pale of depression and uncertainty, Susan is able to say, "perhaps tomorrow will be better, and if not tomorrow, the next day for sure." I am glad she can say that and believe it in the face of such difficulties. How she can be so convincing when she says that is remarkable. It simply shows the depth of her determination, perseverance, and resolve to get better. It truly will happen – I believe her.

Work is crazy—too much, no time and no support; it is hard to work in such an environment. I need to really break away and be an independent contractor.

Still facing the CAT scan on April 2. I know we are both wondering what if the abscess is back, not resolved—what's next? All questions we are afraid to ask each other so we do not discuss the matter. Just the same, I am sure we both think about it. The upcoming CAT scan is constantly on our minds.

Matthew is full-time work; there is hardly time for anything else. I know it sounds like I am surprised by this fact. Susan and I talked about how we just have to do things even if it is just as simple as packing up and going for a ride. Susan is in the house all week and it is hard to be in on the weekends as well. This upcoming weekend, we are going to the ballet; should be an experience to get up and organized so we can drop Matthew off and be downtown in time for the performance.

We joke sometimes about the stroke being an unbelievable nightmare. The more we joke the deeper the pain. I am not sure we could survive if we didn't laugh and use dark humor to get us through. This is us. Might as well laugh your way along the journey. Better than the alternative.

An example is in order, when Susan was in rehab she was allowed a day pass so we went over to the Magnificent Mile, the great shopping area in Chicago. Since this was one of our first "outings" we had to deal with the cold, snow, and slush that provide a winter challenge, but an extreme challenge to someone in a wheelchair. If I had a plow on the front of the wheelchair I could have made a few bucks cleaning sidewalks.

We noticed how few people were physically disabled, in a chair, or using a cane. So, it is not an exaggeration to say we stood out.

While out, Susan wanted to stop at Tiffany's to get a replacement charm for the one Melinda had bought her that held Matthew's picture—the one that was thrown out when Susan's hospital gown was changed.

When she returned to her room at rehab carrying the distinctive teal colored Tiffany bag, Susan's nurse said, "I see you got a little something for yourself". Susan said "Yes, just a little thing."

The nurse then said, "I bet it cost an arm and a leg," to which Susan replied, "I already lost an arm and a leg."

The nurse couldn't believe what she had said, or Susan's quick retort. The nurse was very embarrassed and very apologetic. To Susan it was a good laugh. She told the nurse, "No big deal, don't worry about it." She and I had a great laugh.

I'm going out of town Thursday night. Joyce is coming to stay overnight and I should be back by late Friday afternoon, so that there will be the least possible disruption. It's a project to get organized and arrange who is doing what. I have to shop a few days ahead so that there is food in the house for Matthew and everyone else while I'm away. Now that sounds simple enough, but it's the idea of having to think about all these things and do them all that is a challenge.

On to other things—will write later.

March 18 - Thursday: 8:05 a.m.

Now is quiet time and a chance to do some writing before Matthew gets up for the second time and Susan gets up for the day.

The meeting with Dr. Joanne Smith went very well. She is extremely kind and thoughtful, as well as thorough. She identified Susan's shoulder and hip as muscle tears. Medications, time and ice are the only treatments available.

X-rays and blood work all look okay. The white count hasn't gone up yet, but "it takes time" according to Dr. Smith. While saying Susan looked great, she pointed out that Susan is a muscular mess. The stroke and paralysis and a fall onto her left shoulder have all contributed to her having aches and pains that are bearable, but bothersome. As the body adjusts to the new configuration of what is doable, the muscles and joints will eventually settle down, meaning less pain and discomfort.

While I left to arrange for the next appointment, Susan and Dr. Smith started talking about her feelings of depression, etc.—what to do; what can be done? Dr. Smith was very kind and considerate. Let me summarize what she discussed with Susan.

"It will take time—quite a bit of time—but things will improve. While I don't know what you or others go through on a personal level, I can tell you that the people who have disabilities and get on with their lives (make it to the other side) come to see their struggle as a nuisance and a bother. Somehow they have come to accept a meaning to their life, a reason for going on. That's the challenge—to find meaning and worth.

"Your need to realize that you were critically ill twice and almost died—could have very easily died, but you didn't. The challenge is to find comfort in that and the meaning and value you can make of it.

"Most recovery is on a personal and a spiritual plane. There is the physical challenge or limitation, but the greater challenge is to find the necessary meaning and value that makes you want to go on." Then Dr. Smith said to me:

"For Susan, she is mourning who she was and the fact that, in some ways, she won't be like that

186

*ever again, but that she can become a productive
person. Not knowing the future and/or the
limitations makes everything scary and unsettling. In
that context of what was or what might be, there is
the reality of what is! The daily challenges, joys,
struggles, heartaches, and fears confront all of us.
Susan and her present limitations have to meet the
challenges ahead and then she has to move on.*

*"Remarkably, she is doing great at meeting
this challenge. I say remarkably, because of the
overwhelming nature of the events and circumstances
she has had to confront. Some moments, some days
are not as good as others. Yet, by the same token, they
are not as bad either. It is finding the strength to
meet this ongoing stream of challenges that is the true
miracle. This disability does not go away, it truly is
a nightmare. Yet, you are forced to confront this fact
at every turn. Whether you want to or not, feel tired
or rested, are up for it or not, the challenge presents
itself. Being ready, prepared and eager to meet these
challenges, whether or not you succeed or fail is the
real test. They have to be met—you just have to be
ready to meet them."*

An interesting take, it's the journey and the value of
making the journey, not where it ends that is important.

I'm out of town overnight to give a talk in New York on
Friday. I had to organize and coordinate quite a few people in
order to leave.

Maria comes in late. My mom and Sally (a long time
friend of my Mom's) are coming over in case Maria can't be back
on time. I leave at noon. Amy will come around 6:00 p.m., so
Maria can leave and stay until Joyce arrives in the evening for the
overnight.

Sort of the same cast of characters on Friday, until I come
back about 5:30 p.m.

Better get on with the chores. I feel a bit rested after the previous day when I had only three hours of sleep. I walked the dog and Matthew cooperated last night, so all-in-all a decent night's sleep. Got up at 4:10 a.m. and have been at it since. On to other things.

March 21 - Sunday: 6:47 a.m.

I got up about 3:30 a.m., and then for good at about 4:30 a.m. Matthew was soaked and had to be changed. Plus, he was hungry. He went back to bed about 5:15 a.m. and I stayed up. Took Hans out, did the dishes, made bottles, read the paper, and straightened up the house. Lots to do and might as well do it when there is a break.

My mother and Sally were going to come out and watch Matthew until Maria arrived about 1:00 p.m. In essence, they'd be here until Maria came and I was off to the airport.

My sister, Betty, called. Mother was having pains again and they were worse than the day before. Bobbie, my other sister, was going in to pick her up and take her to the hospital. "Go to New York, we'll call Susan and let her know what is happening," said my sister.

So, at 8:30 a.m. last Thursday, March 18, 1993, Susan's Mother and Dad were on their way downtown for blood work (surgery was scheduled for her Mom the next day). Matthew is crying and I have to pack (if I go). Bobbie is on the way to get Mother who is going to the ER at the hospital.

Like the phrase says, "If you think it can't get worse, wait." Called around and found out that Millie and Harry had plans, Dora was already out, Amy couldn't leave any earlier from school, and Viola and Otto are downtown. So, Eileen (from work) volunteered to stay for a few hours.

I left and worried the whole time I was gone. My Mom was admitted with a blood clot in her lungs. Testing discovered a minor blockage in her leg and an aortic aneurysm.

Susan's mother came through the spinal surgery real well (she's 75 this summer), but she is running a fever and we are hoping it's not anything serious like an infection or something.

The talk went well in New York. The audience was receptive to the ideas and remarks I made. I hope they have me back.

While there, I wondered about home: Susan, Matthew, the mothers, etc. I just can't leave and not think about them. I have to depend on people to help and that's difficult. Joyce, Susan's sister-in-law, who stayed overnight, was suppose to get to our house at 7:00 p.m., but never made it until 8:45 p.m. Good thing Amy could stay as long as she did.

I changed my return flight as soon as I got to New York so that I could arrive home a little earlier. I made it home by 3:00 p.m. What a rush! Worried about migraines, but none occurred. Took the medicine just to be sure.

March 28 - Sunday: 2:50 p.m.

Time marches on, but little changes. It feels like we are stuck in the same maze. We spend considerable time "walking" but going nowhere. It is still a real struggle for Susan and an overwhelming sense of things to do for me. Whatever we do, it takes so much longer, but that's the way it is, so as the saying goes, "shut up and go with the flow."

Both mothers were discharged from the hospital yesterday. My mother's clot is almost resolved and Susan's mother is feeling fine after major neck and spine surgery.

It is quite a schedule to visit both Moms. It's hard to find time to visit my Mom, so I just went into the city to see her today.

Susan so wanted to get downtown to see her Mom, but she has been too tired. The last few days, Susan has had almost a constant headache that gets worse at times. She's not too worried, because she doesn't have other symptoms like dizziness, fever, etc. I don't care, it still worries me. Excedrin, or Advil, doesn't seem to help. She can take two every three to four hours and there is no real relief. At least today the headache doesn't appear to be as constant or as impairing. I will have to look into this.

Worry. The headache, the shoulder, and this six month window to make the most gains that are likely to be made are fast approaching. All are sources of worry, just depends on which one is prominent at the moment. Headache or not, there is always the lingering feeling of when will the bomb go off again.

Susan and I went to the grocery store last night. Saturday at 7:00 - 8:00 p.m., there is nobody in the store. First time she has been in a food store in five months. Towards the end of her pregnancy, she didn't shop as much because she was tired and sick.

What an experience! She used her chair and tried to sit-walk around the store, but after five minutes she realized that wouldn't work. If she kept doing that she would have a groin pull for sure. So I pushed and she led, while I dragged the grocery cart along with us. Not the easiest act to juggle, but we got through it with only minor problems. Clearly, late night Saturday is the preferred time of day versus early on during the weekend. This is something we will learn; what days and times are best to do what? We need to avoid crowds so she can see more.

March 31 - Wednesday: 4:50 a.m.

I was up at 12:30 and 1:30 a.m. with Matthew; 3:30 a.m. with our dog, Hans; 4:00 a.m. with Matthew; and then decided to stay up. It was just one of those nights. It will be time to feed Matthew soon, so might as well stay up. It's worse to fall back to sleep and then have to get up again. It should be an interesting day.

I arrived home early yesterday and was determined to help Susan clean up and get outside for a walk. To my surprise, she was outside walking with Lois, the physical therapist. Susan did very well—on her feet for an hour walking outside in the driveway and then on the sidewalk around the house. Good for her! It's a big start and she will keep after it. Our goal is to walk around the park which is across from our house. We used to walk our dog all the time in the park and Susan walked the park for exercise while she was pregnant. No matter how long it takes or how many breaks are needed. She is determined to walk it again.

I wanted to take her and Matthew for a walk, but by the time the shower was over and she got dressed, it had cooled off, so I took Matthew and Hans. It was very hard leaving her at home while I am outside with the baby. It was her plan to take him for walks not to see me do it. She looked out the side door to see how Matthew looked in his buggy and then rolled back into the kitchen and cried. We would have walked forever—everywhere—to get out and enjoy the weather, take Hans and give Matthew fresh air. That's all changed, but we are still going to figure out a way to do it. We are still going to take our walks; Matthew may be walking with us, but who cares. Later, if not sooner, we are going to do this.

Susan continues to have headaches which don't seem as bad as the past weekend. Still, she takes Advil multiple times a day. This Friday is CAT scan day. We are real hopeful that all is okay and we can get on with life. After all her walking, her leg was tired last night, but it's good she can push herself and do the walking. No problem with being tired after working so hard.

There are still quite a few things to do around the house and no real time to do them. On weekends, it's impossible to do anything because of Susan's schedule and Matthew. Same is true at night. Most evenings, it's one thing after another until bedtime. We'll have to figure out what can be changed so that it can get easier, although I'm not real confident that will happen soon. Nevertheless, things are OK for now and I am sure new schedules will evolve over time.

I will try and start running in the morning. I'll take Hans with and we can go around the park a few times while Matthew sleeps, or after he is fed and is back in bed. I will do it before Susan gets up.

I'm ready for a nap. Guess I'll clean up while things are still quiet. Once it starts, there is no choice—Matthew will be up and he will want to eat.

April 6 - Tuesday: 7:03 a.m.

The April 2 CAT scan post one month off medications has come and gone. Results are excellent. Abscess continues to reduce. In fact, it is substantially reduced from the last scan. May 7 is the next date and by then it (the abscess) should be a scar line (a calcified strip); meaning it has healed.

The "bad news" is that Susan has to adjust to a substantial disability that will not likely get any better. She is and will be significantly disabled. How much beyond her present capacity she can regain is uncertain. But for sure, the expectation at present is very little progress beyond the current capabilities. So what! She has done remarkably well with what she has been forced to confront. If this is as good as it gets – so be it. Remember "Susan may never walk"- well look at her progress now; there are more gains to come.

As Dr. Fernandez put it, the tissue is gone or damaged and not replaceable. "You need to realize that and learn to adapt to your abilities and limitations. Time to get on with life."

That's a great phrase, "learn to adapt." What does that mean? How do you come to accept yourself as someone less than you were or wanted to be, and be faced daily with countless reminders as to what you can't do (the things you could) and what you can do (but not like you used to do them)? Clearly it is easy for Dr. Fernandez to suggest moving on when he doesn't have to confront such challenges.

Susan is sad, just very sad—who wouldn't be by Dr. Fernandez's comments? While at times she will and will not admit to being depressed, it is obvious that she is. Her affect is blunt, no appetite, no interest in things, not caring to shower for a few days, feeling real tired all the time. Individually, any one issue is a concern; collectively, it is a very serious matter.

We try and talk about these things all the time. One issue she has privately struggled with is the decision of, "Would she really go through this again to have Matthew? Was it worth it?" Knowing what she knows would she have become pregnant?

I tried to point out that this was the wrong question. She never would have gotten pregnant knowing this outcome. Who in their right mind would say this is all worth it. **It isn't!**

Having said that, Matthew is precious—but Matthew is not the issue. The pregnancy was difficult, but she delivered and survived. The care (or lack of it) post delivery almost killed her. That is the issue.

I think this conversation was key. For a while she has been feeling guilty because she would never have become pregnant knowing this would be the outcome. Exactly! I agreed. To think otherwise is nonsense. Not willing to become pregnant knowing the outcome does not mean she loves Matthew any less. It is not Matthew; she survived having Matthew. The failure of adequate care post-delivery is the issue. Those are matters the lawyers are reviewing. It was good to clarify her feelings. Maybe this will help.

April 10 - Friday: 7:20 a.m.

I would have thought that by now, I would have settled into a routine. Not likely. I have been fooling myself into believing one day soon things will change. Change how – I don't even know. Just change. But it just doesn't end. Was up at 2:30, 3:15 and 4:40 a.m. with either the dog or Matthew. I stayed up at 4:40 a.m. and Matthew reawakened at 6:00 a.m. This lack of sleep and freedom, plus countless numbers of things to do adds to everything else. There is no sense of going forward. I just don't want to drown. Trying to keep my (collectively, our) heads above water is the goal.

I went to rehab with Susan to see Dr. Smith on Thursday. Joanne was very encouraging and believes there has been good progress. Susan expected more to occur. Not as pessimistic as Dr. Fernandez, but we will see. Susan had an evaluation from Paula (the PT at rehab) and Paula is impressed by the great progress already made and encouraged by both Susan's walking and leg movements versus how she was walking two months ago. This impresses everyone at rehab. We purchased an electrical stimulation machine to help retrain and fire up her muscles. We hope to achieve normal functioning in the leg and arm over the next month or so with this type of treatment, which attempts to retrain her muscles using focused electrical stimulation.

Susan still struggles with her losses; what the stroke has done to her and her inability to be Matthew's mother the way she would like to be is a constant reality. She sees herself as a "bystander"—not really special in his life, because she is not the focal caregiver or comforter for him.

193

In spite of all the effort she makes to do everything she can, she doesn't give herself enough credit for what she accomplishes. She feels there is always far more that she could/should be doing. This gap between what she wishes she could do and what she can actually do results in her feeling like she is missing the mark. Susan has lost herself, the chance to be a mother, and experiences that only the future knows will occur. A very difficult reality to confront.

Susan has to stop comparing herself to what she would have done and used to do and concentrate on what she can do as the standard. There is no other way. Easier said than done. She is what she is and that is the mark. Using the past as the benchmark is unrealistic and not helpful. Starting from not being able to roll over in bed to what she has accomplished now represents tremendous progress. Will it be enough to satisfy her? Absolutely not! That is why she is Susan and I love her so. Susan will continue to fight to regain her old self.

We went to see the Easter Bunny at the mall, Susan, Matthew and I (chair and stroller, plus his bag). The trip was enjoyable. We had a great time! Matthew cooperated and we actually got decent pictures. At least we tried to get out on our own and see what we could do. It went very well. This is a start. We will have to do more of these types of "outings or field trips" as Susan calls them. That is her cynical way of referring to these "staged" trips. In spite of this "field trip" mentality, she enjoys any opportunity to leave home.

We also took Matthew for his first restaurant meal. Not that he was going to eat, but Susan and I would attempt to consume our food quickly as he watched – quietly watched. Over to Market Square (a small strip mall in town) we went and, by and large, he did okay. He wasn't happy being in the car seat, so I held him while eating which didn't help him too much. We were just able to finish our meal when he started crying. So, I'd have to call that a success. At least we stayed and could finish the meal, in record time I should add.

We have set Matthew's Christening date for April 25, 1993, which is in two weeks. A lot to do in the house: paint, clean rugs and drapes, etc. I am not sure it can all get done or what we will do. We'll have to see. Right now, we are trying to plan the event. Haven't sent out invitations, so you know we are running late. Perhaps we will call people. Just might be easier.

We plan to have caterers do the event at our house. That should work. We will have to see how it goes. Not enough time and hands to get everything done, but I'm sure it will work out in the end. I have also considered going to a local restaurant—which may be the best option of all.

Work is still work. We have some outside business opportunities and are trying to become an independent consulting firm. All represent challenges to the spirit, let alone the workload and the stuff at home, but I am up for it because Susan is such an example of determination. She just keeps going in spite of obstacles. A lesson we could all learn.

I am trying to figure out some time to do something for me, like exercise. I haven't done any in six months. Running in the morning with the dog was a good idea, but I just could not fit it in. Sooner or later, I'll drop dead, plus I've gained weight due to eating. So, when I'm in the coffin no one will say he "looked healthy." Rather, "he was fat, so it wasn't really unexpected." I will have to come up with some type of exercise plan.

Matthew is awake and just had his morning shit—or should I say, bowel movement. We're off to a good start already. Plan to go by Pat's (Susan's sister-in-law by marriage) tomorrow. It will take forever to haul all his stuff, including a playpen where he can nap. I'll start packing now so we can be ready by tomorrow.

On top of all this, I had an infected toenail on my big toe removed. The Novocaine shot didn't work because of the infection, so I just held on to the arms of the chair while he cut stuff out. The doctor said the throbbing will let up today and I can walk around with less pain. Not sure when I will be able to wear a shoe again – maybe clown shoes will work.

Easter Sunday, April 11: 8:55 a.m.

A few quiet moments, so I thought I'd write. Susan, Matthew and Hans are sleeping. I've done wash, dishes, taken out the trash, straightened up the house, and put away stuff.

Yesterday, I lost it. I broke the glass in a frame Susan had purchased. I was trying to get everyone and everything in the house after picking up Matthew from Betty, my sister.

Susan and I went to Woodfield and Matthew stayed at Betty's. We did shopping and errands. We returned items and bought a few things.

By the time we got home at 6:00 p.m. with Matthew, he was insane. I was getting everything out of the car and dropped the package with the picture frame, and broke the glass. That set me off.

In short, I said I was losing my mind. I just had to do something (anything) for me. All the responsibilities and pressures are too much. I just have to figure out a way of doing something, anything, sometimes, once in awhile.

Susan became upset. I tried to explain this had nothing to do with her. I just had to figure out how to do something. Well there is no way I can think of; there just isn't. There is barely time for the things that have to get done, let alone trying to schedule "free time." I'm working at a full-time pace, so it is hard to figure out how I could exercise at work. I usually eat at the desk or work through lunch, or eat in the car driving downtown to an appointment.

Between Susan, Matthew, the dog, the house, all need something and I'm the primary one to do it.

We didn't even have time to put on the electrical simulation pack to work her arm and leg muscles. Today is Easter and I'd rather nap than spend five hours at Pat's chatting.

So we will see what today brings.

May 2- Sunday: 5:10 a.m.

I continue to rise early in the morning. Matthew still gets up; maybe he needs more food or something. Whatever, he is up early as usual.

Obviously, it's been awhile since I have written anything in this book. Susan, Matthew and time are the realities that occupy my day. Plus interest. I didn't know if I wanted to keep talking about things—sometimes it's painful enough to live them; rethinking and writing them out just replays the pain. I am also tired of my complaining about having no time, being overwhelmed, being at the end of my rope. Too much whining and complaining. I should just shut up.

Matthew will be six months old in a few days. Time in that regard has passed quickly. He is doing well and is a lot of fun. All-in-all he is very good and very happy. We took him for his six-month pictures yesterday—should turn out cute. Susan had a couple of outfits for him, plus we got a picture with mom and Matthew that will be nice.

Susan has been working hard with the new occupational and physical therapists and is walking much better, but her arm and shoulder are still problems. I'm not sure what can be done.

She's depressed. I know I use the word depressed or depression frequently. I'm not sure what it is other than profound sadness and a sense of loss. At times it is more apparent than at others. I should also note that I am not exactly Mr. Sunshine. Together we make a lovely couple. Back to the issue of sadness. It's to the point of maybe doing something about it. She has been very tired and for good reason, but these waves of sadness seem to come over her. We have talked about a variety of things (hopes and fears), and she is facing more than half of her life being permanently disabled (if she lives that long as she likes to point out), perhaps it is time to talk to a professional. If I am suggesting it, that gives you a sense of how concerned I am. The physical problems have been the focus with little time to concentrate on feelings. Now seems to be the time. It is not that the idea of counseling has not come up for discussion before. Perhaps now is the time.

How much functionality will she get back—independence, if any—care for Matthew—a life? Aside from Matthew who is a full-time job, Susan looks at catalogues most of the day. There has to be more to life than catalogues. But given her headaches and assorted pains, can she really focus on anything.? Is she able to concentrate? Catalogues help her keep in touch with the outside world since she rarely goes out. Most of the time she flips through the pages. She is in quite a bit of pain so I wonder if she can actually look at these products.

We try to get out shopping, or eating, but she is uncomfortable in public. She doesn't like people looking at her. She feels like a freak. While all this is probably true, what are we going to do about it—stay home forever? Hide?

Even the weather is becoming nicer. But it is not easy to get everyone outside at the same time. Susan still can't walk any distance, so taking Matthew for a walk (like we had always planned) is not possible. We need to find a way to take him along in the wheelchair. He could ride in a jump seat like on the back of a bike or something like that. Just have to find someone who can make this—or make this sort of adaptive equipment that can fit on the front of the wheelchair so I can push both of them. I'll design it. Perhaps rehab can make it.

I'm tired. On the weekends everything that needs to get done, I do. With little sleep, I am exhausted by 8:00 p.m. Also, there is no chance to do the little things like cut the grass, wash the car, clean the garage, or go shopping. We have both lost our independence and freedom.

Work is work. I have more contracts on line and have been writing grants to fund our work. What happens—happens, but I think we'll be all right. There is little we can do, so we just do what we can and let the rest happen.

I need to take some time off to do things around the house and for Susan and me to do things together. In the next month or so, I'll take off a week. There are vacation days banked and I should use them or I will lose them.

I know there has been a lot of things happening since I last wrote and it's hard to recall them all. I was talking to a colleague at work the other day about "can't wait 'til _____." I couldn't complete the statement. Things are never going to be what they were and we just go from there. No sense of remembering or comparing, because the only game now is progressing and getting on. You have to keep moving—there is no other choice. Either you keep moving or you become a target. The basic question is the direction of the movement. Far too often is seems we are stuck going sideways. The same issues over and over. It is extremely important to see and feel like you are making progress.

June 11 - Friday: 5:45 a.m.

It's been a long time since I've recorded anything. Days and weeks have passed and yet things are unchanged. Not that anyone expected any real change. You hope, but you also get tired of hoping. Once you feel tired of hoping against hope, you just say to yourself: "Today is what it is, tomorrow is another opportunity." I have to force myself into believing this just to keep going.

It's very painful; very draining; very depressing. This is our life and it's a struggle; wouldn't have it any other way, but the struggle takes its toll.

How Susan goes on each day is a miracle in itself. All of what she had, could do, would do is gone. She can't do what she wants, when she wants to. Choice, freedom, autonomy, independence, plans—name anything, and it has been changed forever.

A little more than seven months have passed. At times, everything has occurred so quickly that it feels like seven days. At other times, it is hard to remember what life was like before the bleed. It's like things have always been this way.

The lawyer called—the case is gray and not clear cut. They only want a sure thing. They haven't rejected the case, but we are looking into a second opinion. We talked to Dr. Smith as to what her thoughts were. She was helpful and very thoughtful. In effect, she wonders what happened. What order was there to care for Susan? What wasn't done that could have been done? I felt very encouraged that things weren't done right after the talk with Dr. Smith. It is comforting to know that Susan and I are not the only ones who believe proper care was not provided. And if proper care was provided, the bleed would not have occurred. In short, what happened never should have happened. It is very difficult to accept this.

Work is a real mess and it's hard to say what will happen. How my team and I will work at the new research institute in the health system is a whole other matter. A job is a job. It pays the bills, but I had hoped to be elsewhere and not in this position at my age. May take my severance package and move on – funny how we are all supposed to "move on." Neither of us has a clue as to what this phrase means or where we should "move on" to.

Matthew is wonderful! He is a joy! He is always smiling and laughing and having a great time. He enjoys life and is basically a real good baby. He has his moments and gas can be a problem, but nothing else. Growing, healthy, lots of fun—and work.

Maria is still helping us. I know the situation is extremely difficult for Susan, but in some ways Maria has made things a lot easier. Easier for me, probably far more difficult for Susan. I could still be looking and going through a host of ladies in order to find the one that would work out the best. But all things considered, she is very loving and kind to Susan and Matthew – of course that is my perspective. I am not the one receiving her help, my guess is Susan has an entirely different viewpoint.

Susan's health is not right. Some type of blood problem (low white blood cells) that leaves her extremely tired has emerged. The heavy and long term treatment of the bleed/infection by antibodies has caused her white blood cells to decline, leaving her at greater risk for infection. It is hard for her to do anything without getting fatigued. Neutropenia is the condition. The bone marrow is affected. There is talk of a bone marrow biopsy. Are they kidding?

Susan's shoulder is somewhat better, but still sore and it bothers her. Not much use of her left arm, although she is regaining tone and perhaps only time will tell (see how hope creeps in).

It seems like Susan sees doctors and/or therapists all the time. Four times a week times for OT and PT, plus at least monthly for both Drs. Smith and Biller, along with monthly CAT scans. Now we have a need for a new OB/Gyn and perhaps a blood doctor to look into bone marrow problems. In spite of all this, Susan has made great progress in her walking. She can bend her knee and point the toes up which, in effect, make it easier to walk and this does not stress her hamstring or groin.

The experience at times is still overwhelming. Sounds like I thought it would be over quickly. The last few days, I don't think I can do one more thing. Everywhere I turn there is something to do, and the cycle repeats itself. I've gained weight because I have stopped exercising (of any kind). I barely have time to do what has to be done, let alone free time for myself. That's a real joke—make time for myself—like it's even possible. Like I can even think about what I would like to do. Guess I didn't take my advice and just shut up. I never thought I could be such a complainer. At least it's to myself and no one else.

Quiet tonight. Susan is out for dinner with former associates who worked with her at Lutheran General Hospital. Matthew went down early because he hardly slept all day. My Mother went shopping with Betty and John. So here I am trying to stay awake so I can continue writing. Impossible. A losing cause.

Chapter 8

TOUGH CHOICES

"It is faith in something and enthusiasm for something that makes life worth living."

- Oliver Wendell Holmes

November 1997

The daily diary, as you can tell from the entry dates are not daily. Not surprisingly, the idea of daily entries became unmanageable. I stopped writing in June of 1993. I am aware that events captured in the moment can have a different feel then when they are recalled and told. "Feel" is the correct word. Feelings experienced as you write about them give events life. Nevertheless, having lived these events prevents me from ever forgetting what they felt like. What has happened in our lives will always be remembered. Not sure if that is good or bad. It just is.

As I write today (10/28/97) Susan is approaching the 5th anniversary of the "event" – as it has been called. Like it is a grand occasion that needs remembering. The daily reminders make it impossible to forget, even if we wanted to. In many ways the five years do not feel like five years and in other ways it is hard to remember our lives before the stroke.

For me, each time the anniversary of her stroke approaches, the tension, anger, the reliving of "what ifs" build up. The thoughts about what happened are never far from my consciousness and I would expect it is the same or probably more intense for Susan. Yet, around the date when the stroke occurred there is an intense rawness to these feelings; these feelings are magnified. I know what is coming and would give anything to go back, give Susan a second chance.

Added to these feelings of loss, sadness, edginess, is the birthday of our son. How ironic we celebrate Matthew's birth only to realize the catastrophic event that followed.

Matthew turned five on November 6, 1997 and I turned 53 on the 5th anniversary of the bleed/stroke. Nothing to really celebrate. I was never big on birthdays to begin with, so you could say that what happened has put a damper on having a grand old time. I am not sure Susan feels the same way as I do. I don't think we have ever discussed it.

People and even health care professionals talk about the anniversary event phenomenon. Alcoholics are educated not to feel their recovery is done when the anniversary of the last drink occurs. Be cautious. Don't have a false or exaggerated sense of confidence.

In our case, the day simply brings back a flood of memories that will never be forgotten. It is as if a weight becomes heavier and heavier as the anniversary date approaches. It builds up in the week or so before the anniversary date and then these feelings dissipate quickly, but the build up is a profoundly sad and painful time.

So what has happened since the last entry.

By the beginning of July, 1993, the CAT scans had revealed that the infection, per se, had resolved. What remains is a residual calcified strip which represents the encapsulated materials. The strip, as seen in the films, seems about four inches long. It doesn't look like much except it can best be described as a very thin chalk line. There is this white, thin line that is surrounded by darkness as seen on the CAT scan film. Looks like a hairline fracture on the right side of her skull.

At the time no one mentioned to either of us the significance of this calcified strip. We have since come to learn that the strip is the epi-center of seizure development.

Blood testing, labs, rehab visits, OT/PT sessions, doctor visits, have come to dominate our life. Services are needed and Susan's health has to be monitored. But over time these visits have tailed off.

At this point everything, everything continues to be a challenge and a struggle. Susan still needs help and her ability to care for Matthew is limited. However, in spite of her own health issues or the tiredness or the aches and pains, Matthew was and still is her priority. When he was young, she did what she could or supervised what was being done as best as she could. Either way, the personal sorrow and heartache she experienced through her inability to care for Matthew the way she would have wanted to is known only to her. It was difficult for me to see her struggle as she tried to dress him or feed him, yet her determination is not to be denied. What little she could do was inspiring. She was determined to do whatever she could do and then some. This has been her approach since day one and I suspect it will always be her approach to whatever challenge confronts her for the rest of her life.

I recall giving Matthew his baths in our tub. Susan would sit on the toilet seat and watch me wash him, making sure I was thorough. Eventually she figured out that if a towel was placed on the tile floor next to the tub and a towel over the edge of the tub, she could kneel down (with much difficulty) and lean on the tub edge to support herself while she washed Matthew with one hand.

More often than not I was accused of doing things too quickly. I wanted to get the task over with. Why take 30 minutes when I can do it in 10 minutes? I realized (not very quickly I might add) that time was not the issue. The important issue was Susan's involvement. More directly, Susan doing whatever, irrespective of the time it would take. Doing is the word. Observing wasn't good enough. Participating was vital.

With more distance from the event and learning a great deal about preeclampsia, eclampsia and treatment guidelines, we are both convinced that the stroke was preventable. That conclusion doesn't sit well with either of us.

After the January 1993 seizure it was not until July 28, 1993 that Susan experienced her second episode of generalized seizing. It was about 8:00 pm. Matthew was down for the night, and Susan and I were watching some TV. For some reason, I looked over towards her. She was sitting to my left and I saw her left arm rising until it was above her head and she began to turn her body, in a slow, deliberate manner, towards the upraised hand/arm as if to follow it. In doing so she started to turn sideways in the chair.

My first reaction was that Susan was doing some type of exercise, like stretching or that slow movement Chinese form of exercise. I was about to make a sarcastic remark when I realized that Susan was lifting her left arm, the arm that was paralyzed and which could do little if anything. Yet how was this stretching routine possible? She didn't respond to me and when I stood to walk towards her she was drooling and her eyes were fixed, not blinking.

It's a seizure, I thought to myself. She is having a seizure. As I began to grasp what was occurring Susan became very rigid and began slipping off the chair. Efforts to stop her from sliding were unsuccessful. I gently held her head and allowed her to go slowly to the floor. Believing she was safe, but experiencing a medical crisis, I called the paramedics. I decided after I took her to the ER the first time that the first time was going to be the last time I was going to be the paramedic.

My sister came over to watch Matthew while I went with Susan to the ER. I had prepared a one page medical history summary which the paramedics found quite helpful. It allowed everyone involved with her care, to be up to speed on her history and the salient issues quickly. I insisted the ER physician call Dr. Biller before any "CAT scan or neuro-work up would be started." Dr. Biller was able to convince the ER doctor to medicate Susan and after a few hours of monitoring we went home.

Since this second ER visit, over time Susan has had 42 additional ER visits. Since most of these visits are to our community hospital, all (ER staff) know the drill. Even the paramedics know the protocol. Try and stop the seizures with whatever amount of medication is necessary. No need to diagnose, run tests, schedule CATs. Just stop the seizures and we will go home.

Our health care coverage became a source of worry and a major source of aggravation at a time when the last issue we wanted to focus on was our health insurance. Would we lose it or would Susan use up her benefits? In spite of our coverage plan, every time I spoke to one of the insurance company's representatives, I was made to feel like somehow Susan was just wasting health care dollars. During one such call the associate said to me "This stroke is costing the company a lot of money; you (meaning me) are just going to have to pitch in and help out. You can't expect us to be solely responsible for this medical problem."

When I heard their standard complaint I usually responded with "We pay health care premiums precisely for such an event. Neither one of us is happy with the use of this benefit."

But the phrase, "pitch in" caught my attention and immediately elevated my level of anger. "Pitch in" I thought. "What do you want me to do, perform surgery, change the central line, what? Listen, we have health care coverage. You don't need to tell me what I should do. You just pay the bills because that is why we pay premiums. If you have any other bright ideas keep them to yourself." Can you imagine? Pitch in! I couldn't.

This was only the first of many health insurance problems.

Toward September of 1993, the company I worked for was going under. I had a chance to join the research group at the corporate office of the health care system, but every time I and my future boss had a discussion about what my role would be, the move seemed less and less desirable.

Because of my years of employment, I was able to invoke the severance package available to me. From the day of my termination I received one year of salary and health care. After which, COBRA could be available for some period of time.

Given all the constraints around pre-existing conditions, caps or life-time payments, etc. I decided to explore what the health system's HR could do regarding suggestions for future health care coverage.

As luck would have it, I encountered our former HR executive on one of his return visits to where he had worked. He is a kind man. He always asked about Susan. In the course of small talk I mentioned my concern about health insurance after my severance was over.

"What are you talking about (I had mentioned COBRA)? You don't need COBRA, just switch to Susan as the primary insured when your severance is over." I didn't know what to say.

My facial expression must have indicated my confusion. Mr. Peeks continued, "Both of you were employees. You had a family plan. Since Susan is classified as an employee on permanent leave, the hospital is obligated to offer her the option of being insured when your insurance is finished. She has the option to pick up coverage, which is something I would recommend you do."

What a pleasant surprise. I certainly had no idea this was possible, but it made sense. "Call the HR department at the hospital and see what they say. Let me know what they tell you," concluded Mr. Peeks.

I was eager to resolve this matter so I placed a call as soon as I returned to my office. I asked to speak to someone in heath benefits and after hearing my story I was told I would have to speak to the Senior VP of human resources. I had a sense that HR had been prepared to deal with me (why would they immediately direct me to the Senior VP?).

The SVP gets on the phone (not someone I cared for, too much of a rah rah guy). "Hi Bill. I am well aware of your situation (why should he be?) and we have looked at all possibilities and there is really nothing that can be done when your severance ends. COBRA is about it."

Without mentioning Mr. Peeks, I explained what I felt was possible. After a long pause, he responded, "No. What you mentioned is not even remotely possible."

Having learned the hard way that "documentation/get it in writing" is the only way to generate a record I said, "Well, you may be correct, but then again you may be wrong. Just to be on the safe side I want you to send me a letter stating your position that Susan is not able to exercise her option of picking up health insurance when my severance ends." I am faxing you a letter as we speak, requesting such a letter from you. Since you are well aware of our situation and quite familiar with the issues, it should not take you long to send me your response in writing. This is Tuesday, how about by Thursday."

I continued to tell him that "I will have my attorney and the Department of Insurance review your response."

"This is an awful lot of trouble for nothing. What you want is not possible," he said.

"Send me a letter indicating your position," I requested. "I will send a letter to the Illinois Department of Insurance explaining your unwillingness to be helpful."

The next day (Wednesday) a letter from HR was personally delivered to me. I opened it and it read in part "upon further review Susan Filstead is eligible to enroll in the health insurance plan when your severance is over. She has one month to decide if she wishes to enroll and what coverage/plan she wishes to activate."

Very thoughtful of HR. "Upon further review." They knew all along there was an obligation on their part to make insurance available to Susan. Obviously they did not feel a need to meet their obligation. Worse yet, HR clearly misled me and said "all possibilities had been looked at."

So much for HR, or as I refer to them as the "help refused" department. Clearly this Christian institution of healing forgot about truthfulness.

As an aside, because I refused to take the corporate research position and the issue I made about continuing health care coverage through Susan, my severance package was summarily denied. No grounds were given. This denial was counter to the termination policies we had been given when we started at Lutheran General.

Through an attorney I hired, the full year salary severance benefit was eventually restored. Why deny what someone has coming? Why lie about what someone is due? After a stressful battle lasting well over a month, at least these two major issues were resolved. I had income for the next year and health care was set – at least for now. The month long fight to regain my severance and future health coverage was extremely stressful given my wife's health and our financial situation.

Towards the end of August, 1993 another bout of seizures occurred. We returned to the ER. Susan was stabilized and we left as quickly as possible. These seizures, while a concern, did not seem difficult to contain since I assumed (there is a John Travolta movie in which someone comments about assuming the good guy was caught: "assumption is the mother of all XXXX-ups." You can add the word yourself) that seizure medication would take care of the seizures. Logically as that may seem, it was not working in Susan's case.

November 24, 1993

I could not write on the first year anniversary of Susan's stroke (11/7/93), it was just too overwhelmingly sad. It is a sadness that invades your very being. In the week or so before the anniversary I found myself reliving the event. Remembering details, conversations, the weather that day, remembering everything.

On the day of the anniversary, I was up early and sat by myself, merely watching the clock get closer and closer to the time it occurred. I am not sure why I did this. I didn't find it helpful. I reflected on the year since the bleed and wondered what the future years would hold for us. Matthew's crying brought me back to reality.

Susan had planned a huge 1st birthday party with a farm theme. Everyone was to come in blue jeans, denim shirts, and Susan supplied red bandannas. It was a great party! Matthew bounced around to everyone and thoroughly enjoyed himself.

At about the same time, the first law firm we consulted told us, "There is a substantial case here that should be pursued." But not by them. This firm takes only "sure, no doubt cases" and Susan's situation didn't meet the test of a sure thing. So we will seek another firm.

Susan continues to work hard at trying to regain full functioning of her arm and leg. It is this struggle that is the victory. Whether or not a cure for epilepsy can be found or stopping seizures once they begin can be accomplished are uncertain. But her daily determination to push ahead with caring for Matthew or with OT/PT to regain functioning is what matters. To wake-up each morning and begin again to confront the day ahead is remarkable. Her actions are inspirational.

After the first year anniversary (11/7/93) thru the next two years into the Fall of 1995, the seizures escalated. Seizures that occurred every couple of months became every couple of weeks, then every couple of days. Eventually the seizures were occurring multiple times a day and some days practically continuously. Increased seizures meant decreased functioning. More physical and cognitive impairments meant less ability to participate in life. Susan's health was declining and the effort to find some intervention/treatment that could be helpful intensified.

Susan and I became quasi-neurologists. We tried to find out what treatments were available; what new ideas were being discussed; and, in the end, what viable options were available for Susan to try.

During this "search for a treatment" phase we did not feel that there were a limited number of options. While that may have been the case, believing options were available gave us hope. Susan had an intense belief that something would eventually work, something had to, and no way could anyone expect to live life like she was. So the challenge before us was to find the needle in the haystack. The one thing that could reduce or, we hoped, stop the seizure activity became our mission.

The number of drugs, dosage levels, drug combinations and the sequencing of medications are unlimited, or so it seemed. However, we soon gained a perspective which helped us see things for what they were, smoke and mirrors. Most of the medications have similar pharmacological properties. None of them are targeted to a specific type or pattern of epilepsy. Location of the seizure activity also doesn't matter. Patients are simply to take as much as they can tolerate and wait and see. If seizures stop or are modified then the drug is effective. Those who do poorly after two different medications are unlikely to find any drug that will work.

This is the trial and error treatment approach that was in place. Susan only experienced the error. As seizures increased so did this trial and error approach. First one drug, increasing levels of the drug, and then usually another drug was added to the mix. At one point, Susan's pill dish (where she placed the pills she had to take daily) looked more like a dish of leftover M&M's. Lots of colors, shapes, sizes. Too bad it wasn't candy. At least she could have enjoyed it.

This process continued for the better part of 2 ½ years! That's correct. Two and one-half years. You name the drug; she used it and every other one, either alone or in numerous combinations - with no results. The seizures continued unabated.

At some point, Susan began to ask herself what was worse, the possible downside from epilepsy surgery to remove the center(s) of seizure activity or the medications and their debilitating side effects. Clearly the medications were depriving her of any quality of life. Being in a drug fog for days on end makes living difficult and the enjoyment of anything impossible.

All the medications had "side effects" – a rather bland sounding phrase. It implies that in order to get the "benefits" of the drug, the person might have to put up with a side effect – i.e., a bothersome symptom or set of symptoms. People who take anti-epileptic drugs, (AEDs), know that the side effects are very real and very devastating. Confusion, rashes, slowed thinking, you name it, are just some of the side effects that Susan, as well as the millions who take these medications, experience. The short term or immediate consequences of these drugs are bad enough, but then you realize no one is really sure of what the long term complications of these drugs are. How can your brain tolerate being "snowed?"

Take confusion as an example. Not being sure if you did something. Forgetting that you have been told something, even multiple times, is devastating. Multi-tasking; doing more than one thing at a time. These drugs make doing one thing a huge challenge, let alone multi-tasking. Multi-tasking is all but impossible. Add confusion, the "stunned" effect of being drugged and you feel as if you are not totally "present" although you think you are. Emotions, experiences, and your senses are dulled. Clear thinking and awareness of one's surroundings are compromised.

Weight gain, loss of taste, extreme tiredness, tiredness to the point that your bones ache are common – in short, anti-epileptic drugs (AEDs) are a double-edged sword. The main problem is the lack of clarity regarding what type(s) of epilepsy can be treated most effectively by which medications. In fact the phrase "no seizures – no side effects" is the rallying cry of many individuals with epilepsy as well as their families. It is very difficult to live when one doesn't feel she is "here." It is also very difficult for family members to see a shell of the person they knew because the seizures AND the medications rob the individual of her essence.

A concrete example may bring this discussion close to home. One night following her epilepsy brain surgeries (to be discussed in due time) Susan blurted out that "I'm losing my mind. I have not wanted to say anything because you would think I am crazy, but before I go completely crazy, I thought you should know that if this keeps up, I am done."

"What are you talking about? What do you mean, losing your mind?" I responded.

"I have been obsessed with counting things, saying things to myself by emphasizing and counting the syllables in the word. If I try to stop – because crazy or not, I know this isn't too good to be doing, I feel compelled to begin again and to keep on doing it."

Susan continued: "I count the black tile squares in the bathroom when I sit on the toilet. It is to the point where I don't want to go to the bathroom anymore. Signs on the highway I will repeat and break down the words into syllables. Gasoline becomes gas-o-line and I will keep repeating gas-o-line, gas-o-line, gas-o-line."

"The Larry King show – all I see is CNN, that is all I see and I keep saying it to myself. I know it is obsessive-compulsive behavior but a lot of good that does me, I keep doing it. See what I mean."

"I didn't know. We need to figure this out. You can't live like this," I replied.

I looked up the present medication and learned that such behavior can be a side effect of the drug. That and recovering from the trauma of brain surgery seem reasonable explanations for this behavior. One can imagine how surgeries and various medications can impact the brain in ways that lead to unusual behaviors.

The ER visits, hospitalizations for video EEG brain wave monitoring increased over time, all aimed at trying to determine the source of these relentless seizures. The seizures were so frequent that, in short order, this was Susan's life – consumed by constant seizures.

The video-brain monitoring really makes the patient feel like he/she is in a fish bowl. The purpose is to try and correlate the scalp EEG recordings with the streaming video. When the patient experiences a seizure he/she is to push a button which alerts the tech to mark that section of the EEG tape and flag that portion of the video. Anywhere from 25 to 30 electrodes are glued to the person's scalp in a pattern that will allow for brain waves to be picked up from the various regions of the brain. The patient is constantly being videoed and the EEG runs continually. The EEG is marked and so is the video. Staff comes in immediately after the button is pushed. Numerous questions are asked in the hopes of describing and characterizing the seizure activity. The staff can look at these data concurrently in trying to understand the seizure activity.

The flaw in this assessment protocol is that seizures deep in the brain may not register on the EEG. Minor seizure activity may also not register. Therefore, depending on the patient's unique situation, monitoring may or may not record the full range of seizures that are occurring.

About two years after the stroke, Dr. Biller left Northwestern University for Indiana University Medical School in Indianapolis, Indiana. We followed. We would go wherever he went because he was, and still is, the only physician Susan' trusts. During one of our every other month visits, he began to talk very candidly about Susan's situation. He realized that she and I have become quasi-neurologists and understood far more about Susan' situation than most patients know about their own situation. He clearly felt it was important for Susan and me to know what the situation was and what Susan was up against.

"The problem, in brief, is that patients like you rarely survive the stroke you experienced. The stroke did extensive damage to the right side of your brain in a wide area, not just a small-localized spot. Add the infection which has left this calcified strip that crosses two lobes on the right side of your brain.

"There is no protocol for treating you. Patients with such damage do not live, and if they do, they are not as cognitively intact as you are. So it is really impossible to know what to do since we have very little experience in treating patients with the set of problems you present."

The good news is that Susan lived and the bad news is that no one knows what to do to address her problems.

This calcified strip is a major culprit in the on-going seizure activity. It is as if there is a major highway through her brain which blocks all sorts of signals from reading or connecting to other cells on the other side of the highway. This "highway" not only blocks communication between countless numbers of cells, it also acts as a roadway for seizure activity to move along. The term is called "propagate" or "trailing." Seizures find a route to take that has been used by prior seizures. When one cell misfires the cell next door follows suit. It is like a line of domino pieces falling in a chain reaction. It is not clear why a seizure starts in the first place or why it stops. For many, the triggers for starting and stopping are unknown. Clearly, certain experiences like a flashing light or trying to follow movement will initiate a seizure. There are countless other times when Susan is just sitting and a seizure occurs for no apparent reason at all, and just as quickly it stops.

These phenomena of the calcified strip and trailing allow the seizures to manifest themselves in different ways, depending on what component or element of the brain is under attack. For example, Susan's finger can move involuntarily, multiple fingers can move, the wrist can move, the hand can become very tight (tight fist), a sharp pain can occur anywhere on her left side, like being stabbed by a knife. Flashing light can shoot across her field of vision; she can hallucinate, and lose consciousness. This can happen countless times each day. Some days the seizures get on a roll, sort of a life of their own, and status epilepticus, a state of almost constant seizing for 30 or more minutes, occurs. Such a clinical state requires immediate medical attention since respiratory failure is a distinct possibility. Susan has had far too many episodes of status.

During status periods where seizures are on-going, consciousness and breathing can be affected. If standing, one, in all likelihood, will fall. You can imagine the damage caused by falls. Susan has had three horrific falls and lived to talk about them. That no permanent damage to her brain or face was caused by these falls is another miracle. The sound of her head hitting the floor—can't be adequately described. I occasionally replay it in my mind and I become physically ill when I hear "the sound" again.

This is just a small glimpse into the impact of seizures on one's life! The terror such experiences present to the person with the seizures is horrific. When will it start, start again, stop – will it stop? How long should I wait? Wait for what? Can I afford to wait until I take other medications to try and stop the seizures? Maybe the seizures will stop, give them time, how much time? Maybe I can make them stop – as if the secret to stopping is will power. Should I call 911? I'll wait it out, but how long do I dare wait?

A flow of questions, concerns, fears, apprehensions, worries, surround a seizure and what the seizure per se may or may not portend. That is the terrorizing point, "may portend," the uncertainty, the lack of control over one's mind and body, the cumulative consequences of on-going seizures are all considerations that envelopes one's senses as one awaits the next turn of events. The next seizure.

Continual experimentation with new drugs, either alone or in combination, failed to make any inroads into the escalating seizure pattern. phenobarbital, one of the older AEDs, had been the drug of choice, only because it seemed to contain (poorly at best) the seizure activity. As seizures increased so did the phenobarbital dosage.

For well over a year, Susan had a toxic level of phenobarbital, meaning that the blood level indicated the drug was being taken at a level that had toxic effects: labored breathing, concentration problems, sleepiness through the day and extreme tiredness. All of these and related symptoms were magnified as higher dosages of phenobarbital were taken. At some point one wonders if the treatment is more damaging than the disease. In fact, the idea of piling on high dosages of medication proved futile. Susan had phenobarbital levels three times the highest point on the therapeutic range. The seizures didn't stop! Physically – cognitively Susan was worse off.

Due to the extensive damage in Susan's brain (the right hemisphere) she had a collection of different types of seizures. While there are technical names like simple partial, complex partial, Susan's seizures manifested themselves in a variety of ways as I have previously described. Involuntary movements of a finger, multiple fingers, a wrist, hand, arms, leg, were simple partial seizures.

The second major class of seizures affected her consciousness. She was out-of-touch with her surroundings. There could be a loss of consciousness or a simple stare and being non-responsive when her name is called or she is asked to do something.

These altered consciousness states we began to call "drops" because if one occurred, she would literally collapse and fall. No warning that she could identify, but if you watched her you could see her eyes and face take on a vacant look and then she would fall.

For almost eight months Susan lived with this "drop" seizure phenomenon. It was a profound loss of consciousness which affected her ability to stand. Therefore, everywhere that Susan went, I went. Every time she would stand, I would stand right behind her. Susan would take a step and so would I. Susan wondered if there was a "synchronized walking team" competition we could enter. "I'm sure we'd win," she'd say.

Our son Matthew was starting to crawl and walk a bit. Often it was a challenge to catch Susan before she fell, or get Matthew before he touched something that could hurt him before assisting Susan.

The song "Me and My Shadow" became our sick way of attempting to tolerate my intense intrusion into Susan's private space. There were numerous times when by luck I just happened to be there when Susan was falling. If I wasn't there, there would be no way to calculate what damage could have been done.

Once she had just finished showering. There were grab bars in the shower she could hold onto if she felt weak. As she was "backing out" of the tub/shower, I helped her on with her robe and sat down on the edge of the tub. Her back was to me as she combed her hair in the mirror. All of a sudden, without warning, she stopped talking and started to fall backwards. I braced myself and caught her so she didn't fall or hurt herself as she collapsed on my lap. Had I not stayed to talk she would have undoubtedly hit her back and/or head on the side of the tub resulting in horrific injuries. Events such as this happened often. The unpredictableness of these seizures made them that more dangerous. Literally, at any moment something catastrophic could happen.

Whether in the house, outside, or visiting someone, I was always watching. Even with Matthew, I still made sure I had a sense of where Susan was at all times.

Those falling type seizures occurred frequently each day over this eight month period. Their increase in frequency and the potential harm they could cause led to more diagnostic evaluations to try and determine what, if anything, could be done. The only modification to her care was to increase the dosage of phenobarbital which only compounded the problem by decreasing her alertness and capacity to help herself by bracing before she fell.

At this point nothing had worked. All known medications had been tried. Options were limited (wear a helmet so you don't fracture your skull in a fall). Desperate, I decided to craft what I called an "appeal for help" letter which I sent to the top neurologists at the major academic institutions in the United States. The letter is reprinted here so that the reader can gage the desperate nature of the situation.

Approximately 40 letters were mailed. The individuals who were sent this letter were identified through literature searches and citation index searches which listed their publications. I sent out this letter, a summary of her current medical condition, what had been tried, and a summary of the treatment efforts that had already been employed. I also indicated I would be willing to forward x-rays, scans, etc. if such materials would be helpful in rendering an opinion.

> May 6, 1996
> To Whom It May Concern:
> I am taking this extraordinary step of writing this letter soliciting your help on behalf of my wife, Susan Filstead.
> At age 38, Susan had a cerebral hemorrhage (right motor cortex) following the birth of our son (11/07/92). Over the course of the past 3 ½ years, her health has deteriorated and, in spite of extensive efforts to treat her intractable epilepsy, we have exhausted all our health care resources in the Chicagoland area. We feel we have run out of options and trust this letter will give us renewed hope for some medical stability and a chance for Susan to enjoy life again.

We are seeking your assistance or your suggestions for locating someone with expertise in the treatment of what we call "drop," i.e., atonic seizures. Sometime there is an aura, e.g., a noticeable weakness in her left leg, an epigastric sensation or metallic taste in the mouth, but not always. My wife will fall or slump over in a chair and lose consciousness for 15 – 30 seconds. If standing, she will fall to her left (she has left-sided hemiplegia). Afterwards, her left side is very weak (more so than it normally is), she has difficulty walking, and has an intense headache behind her right eye that can last for one to two hours. She experiences four to eight atonic seizures, along with several sensory seizures per day.

We have tried numerous anticonvulsant medications, as well as a surgical intervention to control the epilepsy, but none have been successful. The quality of her life has markedly deteriorated and these ongoing seizures present serious risks from falling, as well as cognitive/mental status changes. We could deal with the consequences of her disability if, somehow, we could manage to control these drop seizures.

At this point, we are desperate and need a break. Hopefully, you or someone you might recommend would be able to offer some hope and options for addressing this debilitating condition. Very few individuals know and/or understand what she has to go through just to get through the day. We have a 3 ½ year old son, at present; it is hard for her to participate in his life. In short, we need a chance to rebuild our life and these drop seizures are a major obstacle to moving forward.

Thanks for your time and consideration.

Sincerely,

William J. Filstead

A total of 15 responses were received. The appeal letter was conceived at a time when hope was rapidly fading. As efforts to control the seizures failed, it become more imperative to do something, to take action, to try and discover some new medication or intervention that held promise. That could work.

In effect that is what hope is – a promise to oneself to try and do something to change the course of events. In doing this, in taking action, one's sense of hope is renewed. The responses we received reaffirmed our belief that others concurred that the situation was untenable and offered us their best suggestions for treating Susan's epilepsy, if nothing else. I sensed that others cared about what had occurred to Susan and offered whatever advice they could.

The letter was conceived because of the rapid decline in Susan's health and her quality of life in the months preceding this appeal for help. By the fall of 1995, her life became practically unlivable because of the devastating nature of the seizures and the toxic impact of phenobarbital. More hospitalizations and ER visits led us to contact a prominent neurologist in the Chicagoland area to get a second opinion (actually this was about opinion number five or six). It was an opportunity for a fresh perspective; it was worth exploring. Perhaps an opinion uncluttered by the past course of treatment failures could provide a suggested future course of treatment.

Various meetings, diagnostic workups, tests, scans, etc., led to a recommendation for epilepsy surgery. We knew this option was a possibility, but never considered this treatment as a viable option for Susan. She had tried to avoid considering more brain surgery, given what it entailed and the extensive nature of the damage to her brain. What would the surgeon cut out? We soon learned that was the wrong question to ask. What would be left of her after these surgeries? This question provides a sense of how dire her situation was.

To say that epilepsy surgery was an option doesn't accurately convey our dismissive stance toward it. The very idea of more brain surgery was inconceivable. The prior brain surgeries were decisions necessitated by a crisis. Susan really did not have a choice. In spite of her debilitating health, and the obvious risk that seizures presented to her cognitive abilities and the real potential for

falling, the idea of epilepsy surgery had been viewed more as a
remote possibility than as a viable option. A possibility but highly
unlikely is how we viewed it.

Susan took the recommendation as a suggestion while I am
sure the recommendation was offered in a more insistent tone.
Susan talked with her doctors and anyone else who would listen.
I'm sure she had many more conversations with herself than she'd
care to admit.

What an "option!" Susan should sign up for not one but
two brain operations. The first would install electrodes/plates on
the surface of her brain to directly monitor and map where the
seizure activity was occurring. The second operation would happen
10 days later – that's correct 10 days after the first surgery, to
retrieve the electrodes and also remove whatever tissue was thought
to be causing the seizures. Two brain surgeries within a span of 10
days.

Two events in the late fall of 1995 pushed Susan into
deciding to have the surgeries. In November, 1995, Susan was
hospitalized due to status – uncontrolled seizures. Status had
become more frequent and terrifying. Since breathing is affected, it
is vital to start oxygen to assist in her breathing and head to the
hospital as quickly as possible.

During this hospitalization the doctor suggested that Susan
should take an excessive amount of phenobarbital. It may sedate
the brain to a point that the pattern of the seizure could be
disrupted. When I first heard this suggestion I thought if you can
sedate the brain isn't the rest of the person sedated or isn't the word
coma used to describe such sedation?

At the point Susan was at, any suggestion would be
considered. Regardless of how implausible it may be, a suggestion
provided a sense of action, of doing something, of attacking the
seizure rather than allowing epilepsy to take over.

For a few weeks, perhaps a month, Susan was on a very
high does of phenobarbital. Her blood level approached 75 when
the therapeutic range is 15 – 40. As one of her doctors put it "if I
took this much phenobarbital I would never, ever wake up." That
description fairly described Susan's condition over this course of

treatment. Getting up, staying up, staying awake, being able to talk, all became formidable tasks. As this point she wasn't taking a drug – she was in a drugged state. The seizures persisted.

Susan was hospitalized in early December 1995, because she was having difficulty staying awake, her breathing was shallow, and she was starting to soil herself. She was approaching a vegetative state.

Only after being beaten into submission by the continuing onslaughts of seizures and the realization that she had no life if she continued to live in "la la land," did Susan reluctantly agree to the epilepsy surgeries.

Having decided to undergo the epilepsy surgeries (a point of clarification, the relentless seizure activity forced her decision), Susan thought it was a wise idea to meet with the neurosurgeon, Dr. Whistler. It seemed like a good idea to meet the person who was going to cut open your head and remove tissue that may play a major role in being who you are. Somehow, common sense told her to clear her head of this high dose medication and schedule an appointment to talk with him. In a call to his office, his secretary indicated: "Dr. Whistler usually doesn't meet with patients prior to the surgery (how odd is that I thought?) but I understand your situation and I will arrange a time for you to see him."

The appointment was scheduled and Susan had her list of questions. "So what is the plan and what possible problems and further losses am I facing?" she asked Dr. Whistler.

> *"Let's start with the obvious," he said.*
> *"Death can happen, has happened, but rarely does.*
> *Infection can occur, and does occur more than we*
> *like, and you have already had one before. You could*
> *lose sight in your left eye, for sure your peripheral*
> *vision will go and maybe hearing on the left-side will*
> *be reduced. Your arm is already paralyzed and your*
> *ability to walk may initially be difficult or you may*
> *be unable to walk at first, like the way you stand and*
> *walk now. The way you are today is about the way*
> *you will be after these surgeries. More or less."*

"What about seizures?" Susan asked.
"Hopefully, we can reduce them, but in all likelihood
not eliminate them. Reducing the frequency should
improve the quality of your life. Any more
questions?" he asked in a tone indicating he was done
talking.

I'm sure Susan would have wanted a person
who was more compassionate or showed more
understanding for the situation she was in, but that
wasn't going to happen. I'm not sure he was capable
of anything more. As I told Susan, "Who cares if he
cares as long as he is good, real good."

As we were about to leave Susan said,
"Thank you for your time. See you in the O.R."
That is an attitude I admire. Bring it on. Let's get
it over with.

Hindsight is wonderful. As simple as it sounded then –
that the seizures had to be monitored and mapped to assist in
deciding how to perform the second surgery, it did not turn out to
be that easy or straight forward. The initial brain surgery to place
the grids was problematic. There was scarring from the prior
surgery and the damage due to the initial bleed itself; tissue had
stuck together and to the skull since the last surgery. The way the
damaged areas had healed made it all the more difficult to insert
and place all the grids that were planned for use in the monitoring
phase of the surgery. Bleeding, excessive bleeding occurred during
this grid placement operation which forced the surgeon to do what
could be done as quickly as possible. Susan and I failed to
comprehend the obvious, that the mapping was only as good as the
grid placements. No grids in certain places meant there were no
readings about that area of the brain. The idea of an incomplete
mapping of the seizure field never occurred to us. Like the story of
the person who drops something on the street and chooses to look
for it under the street light rather than where it fell, I had assumed
that the grids were placed where the seizures were occurring. It

never occurred to me that the mapping of the seizure activity would be either difficult or incomplete. Why are we supposed to know this? Why didn't anyone mention this contingency in the discussions prior to her surgery?

The first epilepsy surgery accomplished what it could. When completed, the part of the skull that is removed to allow for the grids to be placed is loosely replaced so that the wires from the implanted electrodes can be threaded out the back of the head and connected to the EEG machine. I liken the situation to having a pony-tail of wires coming out of your head that are attached to grids that are inside your head. Susan was expected to live like this for the next 10 days or until enough seizure activity readings were obtained so that the information to support the second surgery could be acquired and a plan for the second surgery developed.

Her head was wrapped like a mummy. She had a major headache, which I'm sure we can all appreciate to be a gross underestimate of the pain she was experiencing. It was practically impossible to lay on her back due to this large pony-tail of wires. When she went to the bathroom this entire apparatus of wires, battery pack, IV's, tubes, etc. had to go with. Ten days! That is the expectation. Living life this way for 10 days. If one of the neurosurgeons would have to experience this state, I'm sure a different protocol would be developed. Ten days is next to impossible.

On one of my visits to see Susan following the first surgery, the neurologist who was charting her seizure activity saw me in the family waiting area. He approached and asked if we could talk for a few minutes.

> *"We have been monitoring Susan and,*
> *while we know where many of her seizures originate,*
> *we have not been able to pinpoint the location of the*
> *drop seizures. I'm beginning to wonder if perhaps*
> *these are pseudo-seizures."*

> *"Pseudo seizures – like they don't exist?" I*
said.

"Well that's aboutÖ." I interrupted, *"You are suggesting that since you can't find them, they don't exist. Perhaps, in your mind, that's the case, that they probably don't exist. Are you kidding me? Are you crazy?"*

I continued, "You have determined that if you can't find the origin of the seizure that it doesn't exist. Who the hell do you think you are? Is this the standard of care? If it can't be found it must be psychological? Maybe you placed the grids incorrectly. Maybe the origin of the seizure is deep in the brain and the grids can't pick up the activity because it dissipates before reaching the surface of the brain.

"All the scarring from the bleed, the calcified strip, etc. can't cause seizures? She has been playing a game? You are crazy. Let's get things clear. I don't want to hear the phrase pseudo-seizures used again. I don't want you to say it to Susan or write it down anywhere. Your incompetence is not going to come back to haunt us. Do I make myself clear?" All he could suggest is that the seizures could be psychological. Like Susan gains from falling all the time. Well, maybe someone would, but that someone is not Susan.

"My mistake for bringing it up," he said. *"It won't come up again. We will do more monitoring at the time of the second surgery when the grids are removed to see if additional data can be obtained that will direct the surgery."*

End of discussion.

I couldn't believe this exchange. Pseudo-seizures! Like there are no structural indications of damage that produces seizures. What a joke, unfortunately this "joke" is played on individuals more than one realizes. It is far too easy and convenient to place blame on the patient for failing to produce the data necessary to make a diagnosis. God forbid it could be the physician who fails to find the source of the problem, to understand it or diagnose it correctly.

After almost 10 days, Susan underwent the second craniotomy to remove the grids and resect and transect the sections of the brain determined to be the source of her seizures—or at least this was their best guess as to what tissue to remove given what the grid information revealed.

The neurosurgeon told me, following the second brain surgery, "Your wife is very tough. I think she could be run over by a Mack truck and get up and walk away. She has been through hell a few times; I hope this will be the last trip. I hope the surgery is a success."

Susan was hospitalized from January 7, 1996 through January 18, 1996. She was discharged to home. Her rehab physician was kind enough to come by and do an assessment to see if a rehab course of care was necessary to gain or regain the level of functioning that existed prior to the surgeries. "I'm pleased to say, go home. You are doing remarkably well. I will order home care," said Dr. Smith.

Epilepsy surgeries are barbaric. What other term can describe what is done? Shave your head, cut through the scalp and skull to expose the brain, and then go digging around in the brain so you can insert these grids (thin pieces of encased wires), put it all back together, wait a while, and do it all a second time.

In my way of thinking, the brain is you, it is your essence, your self, it is who you are. Recovery from brain surgery takes time: six to nine months to fully overcome the insult received. Fortunately, Susan avoided an infection and did not develop water on the brain (Hydrocephalus) requiring a shunt to drain it. No serious complications except the impact on her body and the time it takes to regain strength, energy, and functioning. I list these side consequences as if these are minor complications – which they are not.

Remarkably, Susan was able to walk around the house by use of a cane or by holding on to objects, table to counter to chair

to sofa, the day she returned home. She didn't miss a beat. She was
back to where she was prior to these surgeries. PT and OT
returned to try and accelerate the recovery of skills and abilities.
Susan was walking—walking slowly—but walking.

Being away meant reconnecting with Matthew, re-
establishing Mom's expectations and approaches. Even though
Matthew saw Susan while she was hospitalized, I'm not sure what a
3 ½ year old can comprehend except to be frightened by the noises,
lights, and the sight of mom with the wires coming out of the back
of her head. But comprehend he did.

Matthew wanted Susan to take his picture to the hospital,
and also his favorite stuffed animal, Ellie – the Elephant, so she
would not be alone. During one visit he wanted to talk to the
doctor who preformed the surgery. Being very verbal and insistent,
he had a way of imposing his will even at such a young age. The
resident who heard this request said that Dr. Whistler was down
the hall and Matthew could meet him when he passed by. Matthew
would have an opportunity to talk to Dr. Whistler, if Whistler
would stop and talk to him.

Sure enough, that is all Matthew had to hear. I walked
with him down the hallway and pointed out the neurosurgeon, a
large imposing man. Dr. Whistler headed towards us trailed by a
collection of residents, fellows, and students.

As Matthew approached, I introduced Dr. Whistler to
him. Matthew extended his hand, to shake Dr. Whistler's hand
and as he did Matthew said "Are you the doctor who is going to
help my Mommy?"

Dr. Whistler, bent down on one knee so he could almost
be eye to eye with Matthew. "I'm your mother's doctor and I am
going to do all I can to try and make her better." That was fine by
Matthew as he stated, "Good. Thank you," and we turned to go
back to Susan's room where he promptly told Susan that he had
spoken to her doctor and the doctor was going to make her better.
Matthew had a way of conveying the surgeon's words which made
it seem true. Like it was a fact. A given. Mom was impressed, as was
I; later a fellow who was part of the tour group commented he had
not seen Dr. Whistler be "confronted" like he was and for him to

"respond so compassionately." "Dr. Whistler was very impressed by your son." The resident noted for our benefit that "Matthew was not intimidated by Whistler like the rest of us are."

While I was visiting one afternoon following the second surgery, Susan asked the chief resident "What would cause sharp pain on my left side?" "Where did it occur?" the resident asked. "Sometimes my leg or sometimes my arm. It doesn't happen a lot and it could be anywhere on the left side. I even had a sharp pain on my cheek." The resident said, "We call that a sensory seizure," to which Susan simply replied, "Oh." The look on her face said more than the casual. "Oh."

Nothing else had to be said. I looked at her as she did me. The resident left and neither of us said anything for what seemed like an eternity. Neither one of us wanted to say out loud what we were privately thinking. Finally, Susan deadpanned, "a seizure, that's nice." Her remark said more than the words conveyed. Disappointed. Dismayed. Disgusted. Defeated. You pick the word that best describes the feelings of hopelessness that enveloped us upon realizing the surgeries didn't accomplish what had been intended. These surgeries were to reduce or eliminate the seizures. Here Susan was, a few days after her second brain operation in 10 days, and she was experiencing seizures. More distressing, she had never experienced this sensory type of seizure before these surgeries. Not a good beginning nor was this an endorsement for epilepsy surgery. Our strategy was to dismiss these newly experienced sensory seizures – which happened four or five times – as an aberration. Never to occur again, or so we desperately hoped. This would be the last of the seizures rather than the continuation or escalation of the seizure pattern that led up to the surgery. Both of us knew that time would tell.

Well, we didn't have to wait long. Over the next few days Susan experienced the focal-motor seizures which she had before the surgeries – the involuntary movement of a finger, toe, wrist, etc. on the left side of her body. What was different is that these focal-motor seizures were quickly followed by the sensory type seizure. Or vice-versa. Thus, a new seizure-to-seizure pattern had emerged within five days after the second surgery. The feeling of "so what did I do these surgeries for?" occurred frequently.

Susan could walk as she had, but the sight in her left eye was affected. She could only see straight ahead. Her hearing was also diminished. It was clear that the surgeries only resulted in furthering her seizures. Sort of a rush to judgment on my part, but Susan did not disagree with this opinion. The "subpiel transaction," cutting through tissue to leave a slim connection between the areas being transected (cut), simply provides the seizures a one lane highway between the tissue sections.

The surgeries had an impact on the occipital lobe – a source of vision. Within a few days of the second surgery Susan saw flashing lights, fireworks, shooting stars in her left field of vision. Even more disconcerting were the seizures that revealed shadows or what seemed like dark shapes crossing her left eye. These sights were so compelling that she was drawn to them, even turning her head to the left to follow them. Intellectually knowing what was occurring could not prevent Susan from going left. Going left would become a harbinger for a string of debilitating seizures that were sure to follow.

Recovery – not sure that is the best word to describe the long protracted process of trying to heal, regain strength, and return to everyday life after such surgeries - takes time. Any surgery has an impact on a person's physical and psychological status. The anesthetic takes time to clear; the pain medication to deal with pain drains you, and the headache from both surgeries and the seizures are practically debilitating. There is the worry about infection, brain swelling, skull bone fit, and the delay in returning to baseline. All were initially judged to be ok – and we would monitor them at home.

In a follow-up with the neurosurgeon, he was pleased with the technical aspects of the surgery, the lack of complications, and Susan's return to her baseline walking. "I'm sorry we could not eliminate or significantly reduce your seizures. We tried," he said.

"I know you did. Thanks for trying," Susan responded.

Try. Try is the key word. So, the search to find something that could, would, might work starts anew. Try is what she had done and will continue to do.

The early efforts at asserting her motherhood role revealed a host of obstacles, the primary one being individuals, myself included, assuming Susan could not do something and then doing something for either her or Matthew without asking. The "taking over" style of helping.

Asking rather than "assuming and doing" is critical for a person with a disability. No one steps in and takes over for an individual who is not disabled – so why the tendency to take over and run the life of the person with a disability?

I'm sure part of the motivation to take charge is a sincere attempt to be helpful. For some, it is a lack of patience, "I can do it and we will be done with it" attitude. For many it is simply ignorance. They are oblivious to the symbolic meaning of their actions in terms of how the person with a disability is made to feel. Every unwanted or unneeded action by someone for a disabled person reinforces the sense of loss and lack of control the person with the disability feels.

Clearly it is not the act of being helped that crushes one's sense of self-worth, but the meaning of the need to have assistance. Much of our life is composed of symbols, language, objects, and behaviors. The person who has the disability clearly, dearly, wants to retain every last task or skill that he or she can, no matter how long it takes, how well it gets done, or even if it is done the way it used to be. The effort to try and do the task represents an opportunity to regain normalcy. Whether it (the task) is done is unimportant.

For example, Susan can tie her shoe with one hand. She can make the knot-bow. It can take 10 – 15 minutes of determination and effort to accomplish this task. When done, the knot does not function like it had before. It might keep the foot from sliding around in the shoe, and the knot itself may come undone rather quickly. Nevertheless, it was worth it to see her tie her shoe.

I often will say, as we walk downstairs, "next step is a big step." I would never have done this before the stroke. I would not be walking in front of her as she descends the stairs (to break a fall if it would happen) before either. Now it is automatic and it is symbolic of how things have changed.

Back to motherhood. There is the daily struggle for Susan to feel like a mom and to be seen as the Mom by others, as well as Matthew. Nothing is more painful to Susan then to have our son act in a way that makes her feel that her effort was not good enough, or more heart-breakingly, that she isn't the Mom. While not intentional on our son's part, any indication that Susan has fallen below the standard (whatever that is) reinforces her feelings of being inadequate.

Such an exchange does not have to happen often, but whenever it does happen, feelings of self deprecation quickly rise to the surface.

When Matthew was a baby, as soon as he would cry, everyone reacted to comfort him, always ignoring Susan. It is not always clear what to do, should I pick him up if he cried or do I have to ask her first? Sounds petty, but it is such interactions countless times throughout the day, week, month that cumulatively exact a heavy toll on the relationship – the relationship is defined by such countless numbers of encounters.

These issues of parental involvement, participation, decision-making, will occur throughout Matthew's life and will be this way forever. The situations may change, the circumstances might be different, the relationship has and will continue to evolve: "this is not the way I thought it would be," Susan will remark. "The question is, what to do? Do what one can or withdraw and let others decide for our son?" Susan makes every effort to be there for Matthew and be his Mom. It took repeated efforts but eventually Susan succeeded in feeling like she is Matthew's Mom and feeling like others knew and acted towards her as Matthew's Mom. It did not come easy and challenges present themselves everyday, but she is up to the challenge.

Uncertainty. Unpredictability. These are two words that convey part of the terror associated with epilepsy, especially intractable epilepsy. The anxiety when seizures start can be overwhelming. It should be noted that such feelings are normal. Who would not be anxious when the seizures reached a stage where the person does not **know** if the seizures will stop or if they will escalate, necessitating an ER visit?

There is an on-going posturing between two factions that are impacted by epilepsy. These "camps" or "factions" comprise a variety of people with epilepsy, family members, health care professionals and public/social policy shapers.

Group A presents a fairly rosy (seems like a contradiction to me) picture of epilepsy. Great strides are being made, more drugs are available, surgery (especially early in the cycle of seizures) offers hope for some, and there is a quality of life associated with living well with epilepsy (an actual theme to an epilepsy conference).

Group B has a less rosy view of things; they are not pessimistic, but realistic. They act as political activists making the point that epilepsy is a forgotten condition and under- funded. Efforts to contain or control it miss the point that the treatments (be they medication or surgery or both) are often as devastating as the epilepsy and the seizing continues for the 30 to 40 percent of people with intractable epilepsy in spite of these treatment resource interventions. These statements aim to say to all within ear shot, face the fact; current treatment goals are not acceptable. There needs to be a cure.

No seizures. No side effects. A cure is needed. Nothing less will do. Seizures need to be stopped in those who have them and prevented in others who may be at risk to develop epilepsy.

Chapter 9

WHAT WENT WRONG?

"In these matters the only certainty is that nothing is certain."

- Pliny the Elder

The OB/GYN who delivered Matthew stopped by to see Susan the second day post the initial brain surgery in 1992. During the course of small talk Susan or I asked, "How common is this (the stroke following delivery)?" His response was, "I've heard about it, read about it, but have never seen it before."

While in neuro-ICU post surgery the neurologist commented aloud, "They should have been monitoring your blood pressure." Implying to me that they didn't monitor it.

Still in the acute setting a rehab doctor said, "I'm sure you will have a lawyer look into this – a third year medical student would know what to do."

These were very troubling statements, but at the time the only concern was Susan's health – not suing anyone. In fact, our initial reaction to the stroke was "shit happens," assuming that everything was done that could have been done to prevent what happened. There was no thought that anyone failed to do his or her job to provide the best care possible. After all, we were at the premier women's hospital in Chicago.

As Susan moved to rehab and these types of comments continued, we made an appointment to see one of the high profile medical malpractice attorneys in Chicago. I had asked for a copy of her medical record from the hospital and was told I would have to wait a week or so because her case was being reviewed. Having worked in health care and being familiar with hospital procedures, I knew Susan's stroke was certainly being reviewed by the adverse events committee or the high risk committee of the medical center. In short, it was being looked at closely because the hospital, like those who had made comments to us, knew something went wrong, terribly wrong.

Once I obtained a copy of the medical record, and read it multiple times, it became clear to me that Susan had been in a medical crisis, yet nothing had been done to help her.

One thing about the law firm we initially contacted is that they win cases. At their office for an initial appointment, we found a brochure about the firm that indirectly explained their success. The firm receives over 1,000 inquires each year from which 100 cases are evaluated. This culminates in a decision to represent 10 of these 100 cases.

I believe the phrase is "cherry picking." They can pick and choose those cases that are a slam-dunk. Cases where the error is so clearly egregious that no one can deny the mistake and subsequent consequences. The only matter to determine is the amount of the award either through settlement or trial. I recall seeing a paperweight (bronze) on the coffee table in the waiting area of this law firm. It was a reproduction of a settlement check for 25 million dollars, the largest award ever given at that time. So Susan's case, while perhaps having merit, had to also reach this standard of a slam dunk.

After a few meetings, a conference was scheduled with the senior partner who said, "While your case has merit we have decided not to take on your complaint." Translated means "We would probably have to work too hard and it is not worth our time to take it on, considering the easier cases we have waiting in the wing."

The key impression Susan and I formed having reviewed (should I say memorized) Susan's medical record and having the meeting with the lawyers at the firm was: care was not adequately provided and what happened was preventable.

In Illinois, perhaps other states, there is a time limit in which a malpractice suit can be filed. In Susan's situation it is two years. Over the course of the next 18 months we interviewed two other law firms until we selected a firm to represent Susan.

A few points need to be made about malpractice, law and lawyers. While this discussion will be brief it is important to understand how her case proceeded in order to clarify how this process works.

First, in Illinois (all of these remarks are specific to Illinois) an independent physician has to review the potential suit to see if he/she agrees that it has merit. Merit means that a deviation from a standard of care can be reasonably assumed. An individual (on his or her own) can't file a suit for medical malpractice. An independent physician reaches a conclusion that the expected standard of care may not have been met. In any event, something went wrong and the case has merit.

Second, the law is the law and it is not necessarily a process of finding out the truth. What may be legally true may not be morally right or correct. For example, minutes of the hospital committee that reviewed Susan's case cannot be obtained by our lawyers. The phrase "out of reach of the law" means that whatever is said in such meetings cannot be "discovered" by us. Minutes could indicate a gross mistake yet the hospital can chose to plead not guilty. From my biased perspective, if such a hospital committee determined the hospital and/or a doctor was at fault why not do the right thing and admit it? Why pretend to be blameless?

Third, no one seemed to be interested in helping us find out what happened. The doctor and hospital want to protect their own interests and may, in fact, see each other as to blame for the suit. Despite this, it is in their best interest to join forces against us. Other doctors may just not want to get involved and to be seen as taking sides.

Lawyers, theirs and ours, are not without their own baggage. Our attorney's fees represent a percentage of the judgment (if there were one) so there is an inherent conflict of interest in trying to resolve the case in a manner that produces the biggest paycheck for the attorney. The matter of a correct, just, reasonable settlement is always looked at (from the attorney's point of view) as "what is in it for me?" Settlements are often negotiated/agreed to because the attorney's pay day can be assured. A trial removes this certainty.

Fourth, those who testified for the hospital developed selective memory or lied outright. Phrases like, "I can't recall," "As best as I recollect," "I can't be certain," and the favorite "I don't remember," are often used. The extent of witness coaching and preparation prior to testimony is extensive. Thus, phrases like those identified above are difficult to comprehend and, from the defense's perspective, are impossible to refute. The issue is not what one knows, but how much information about the case can these witnesses be made to tell and tell truthfully. It goes without saying that the defense witnesses' remember what helped their position and forgot what would be helpful to us.

Two months prior to the two year deadline for filing the suit, a malpractice suit was filed on Susan's behalf. This would start a five year process of reliving the events of that fateful day, daily, while we tried to live our lives. While we tried to move on, the litigation always brought us back. Hearing the events unfold once or twice is extremely difficult. To have to relive them is to experience the pain caused by these events over and over again until all that one has left is pain – no joy. Just painful memories.

Knowing that a failure in care occurred, at least this is what we believe based on the remarks early on, the opinion of the various law firms, and our reading of the medical record, we believe that what happened didn't have to happen. As this reality sets in, it generates a constellation of feelings, the most prominent of which is anger - anger that borders on rage. Anger magnified by the refusal on the part of the doctor, hospital, or anyone to apologize for what happened. The process of reviewing what could have been done to have prevented the bleed in the first place merely escalates these feelings. Having been told that a "third year medical student" would have known what to do to prevent the bleed makes this event that more difficult to fathom, let alone "accept."

As an aside, the ideas of acceptance for what happened and forgiveness for those who caused the difficulty are complicated issues, complicated for us (me) at least. Irrespective of our Christian values, the fact that no one stood up to accept responsibility or at least to say they were sorry for what occurred makes it extremely difficult to forgive. I guess a person can forgive regardless of what anyone else does. Yet, at a very primitive level, it seems to me that one forgives those who ask for it. Forgiveness is something that should be asked for, not simply given.

The topics of anger, forgiveness, acceptance, etc. are probably a book in their own right. Perhaps when that book is written, I will read it to gain an understanding of what to do about these issues, since they are as raw as when first experienced. I doubt if they will ever, ever be resolved so that I am at peace. Susan's feelings on this matter are even stronger than mine. Death will bring peace a whole lot earlier.

Back to the legal process. The discovery/deposition process is extremely time-consuming which makes it very frustrating. A critical event occurred early on in this process which made everyone wonder.

About a month or so after Susan's bleed, I requested a copy of her medical record. The request was delayed until the record could be located, but eventually we received the 500 plus page document. This record we gave to our attorney. Since this initial record was copied so soon after Susan's discharge, our attorney decided to request a second copy almost two years later. The second copy contained a page of information that had been missing (no one knew this page was missing until the comparative copy was available) from the original copy.

In all these 500 pages the only page missing was the sheet that contained the log of blood pressure readings. This is the place where the on-going BPs are logged throughout the course of care preceding and following the birth. Since this was the only page of the over 500 pages that was different between the two versions, it made us seriously wonder why, if any page was missing, it would be the BP log sheet. An obviously vital document. The BP log readings would allow one to examine the actions taken to treat Susan. What was done (or not done) at various blood pressure readings. The BP readings could be seen as indicators of other processes that must be addressed in order to lower her blood pressure.

The factor that pushes such a case forward towards some conclusion, one way or another, is a trial date. Such a date really doesn't mean anything since postponements, delays due to other trials, holidays, etc. can make the real trial date variable. However, having a trial date does make things happen. In November of 1994 we had no idea that the trial date would be almost 2 ½ years off.

Depositions, interviews with experts and/or those involved with the case: nurses, us, the doctor, etc., are supposed to be sworn statements of what was done, and one's opinion as to what happened. Again, the goal of the hospital and doctor was to put the best spin on the situation, avoid blame, and argue there were no signs or indications anything should have been done differently because nothing indicated that anything but standard care was what Susan received. Ours was the opposite position. Given Susan's situation, something obviously did not go as planned.

Susan wanted to know what happened, especially since physicians who had no vested interest in the case indicated that a failure to monitor and provide treatment caused the stroke. In short, Susan believed she did not receive adequate care. The lack of care resulted in the bleed.

The whole legal process takes years. While time passes you are reliving these past events and trying to figure out how to live with the problems that confront you today.

The legal process makes the event front and center most days. At times it felt like it is the only thing that occurred for days. You are asked to remember, recall, provide detail, review documents, tell your story, read the depositions of others, etc. All of these activities make the day-to-day living even more difficult. The more one reads about what care could have been provided, what actions were or were not taken, and reads the notes in the chart, the more one's sense of anger over the failure to provide proper care grows.

For example, Susan complained of, "The worst headache I have ever had" during the early morning hours of November 7th, the day of the bleed. Nothing was done. Chart notes indicate increased vomiting and decreased urine output, indicating that the body is starting to shut down. No doctor saw her. No medications were tried.

At 8:30 a.m. the morning of the bleed, Susan said to a nurse in the room, "I don't feel right, I have never felt like this before, blurred vision, shooting stars, and I can't feel my arm, please call someone, please."

By 9:00 a.m. according to chart notes, the blood pressure had risen to 220/114. The stroke had occurred. A CT was ordered. A large area of bleeding was identified and she was transported to neuro ICU.

Through the course of the legal process we came to realize that right and wrong are not important matters with respect to the law. Legal procedures, processes, and what can be legally "proven" are all that counts. It is not even a matter of what can be proven. The hospital, doctor, and nurses can lie and that lie somehow becomes a fact. Let me give an example. The night prior to delivery, Susan's blood pressure was elevated and stayed elevated throughout the night and into the next morning. After having been moved from the floor to a labor room the morning of delivery (about 7:00 am), her blood pressure was still elevated, occasionally spiking when contractions would occur.

The nurse, Lori, had difficulty obtaining a valid BP reading because the automated wall-mounted unit was not working properly; it would not allow the BP cuff to inflate. So Lori, knowing that BP monitoring was very important, found an old-fashioned BP unit and said, "I'm going to tell the floor that I need to be here all day. Usually, I have two or three rooms to monitor, but I want to keep a close watch on you; so, it will be just me and you today." In her deposition, to the question:

> Q: How would you describe Susan's pre-delivery BP?
>
> Lori: It was normal, nothing unusual.
>
> Q: Didn't you say to Susan and her husband that you were concerned about her BP and rather than work with two or three patients, you were going to stay with her to monitor her BP?
>
> Lori: No. I was in and out of the room throughout the day and took BP readings like I would for any patient.

As I said, so much for the truth. I often wonder how Lori or the doctor, Dr. Toig, can look in the mirror and live with themselves. That is a burden they will have to deal with each day for the rest of their lives. Susan and I, because of them, have our own issues to deal with for the rest of our lives.

Reading the depositions simply re-enforces the anger and outrage. No one would own up to what was **NOT** done. Another example, the nursing BP sheet that was eventually found revealed that her BP readings were "marginal and would not indicate any need for action" according to their expert witness.

An examination of the BP floor sheet indicates what I consider a remarkable string of identical or nearly identical BP readings over a span of seven hours. The published literature that discusses BP readings and what action that may or may not be taken indicates that this BP reading 190/95 is a signal to be alert to possible trouble. This literature suggests that the medical staff look for other signs/symptoms which might clarify the significance of this reading. In short, what is the big picture, not just this one indicator of medical status.

I used the word "remarkable" to describe the universally consistent set of readings contained on the log. It is remarkable because while these BP readings are on the threshold of concern, Susan's urine output, protein in the urine, and liver functioning were markedly declining. Her organs were shutting down because of the rising BP, but this chart does not reveal a rising BP. Remarkably, in spite of the indication of system failure, which you would think would have a major impact on the BP, the BP was consistent, conveniently consistent. It was stable, never going beyond the threshold which would indicate a need to treat the BP. Thus, the picture in the chart is one of a person who is experiencing organ failure and marked increase of toxins in her blood and urine, yet her blood pressure is stable. In fact, it is the same identical BP reading, 190 over 95, over 8 consecutive readings, over a two hour span of time. Any chance that this is actually the true BP reading? I think not.

I should note from the outset, that my feelings for Susan's attorneys are about the same as my extreme dislike of her doctor. The attorneys, while supposedly working for you (their client), have their own interest as the number one priority because any settlement or verdict that is in Susan's favor is a payday for them. Rather than have the attitude of staying the course to the fullest in the hopes of achieving some semblance of justice, their posture became one of getting something with the least effort because they could count on a payday. Some money with little effort was preferable to putting forth effort, with no guarantee of what the outcome would be.

The question of tort reform has been a hot topic with both Bush Administrations (Bush #1 and Bush #2). The idea to cap a medical malpractice award because doctors can't afford their insurance payment totally misses the issue. If a doctor is repeatedly found guilty or settles malpractice claims, don't let him or her practice. Suspend/revoke the license to practice medicine because of the harm, maybe even death, he/she may have caused. Make him/her pay a very high premium due to the way he/she practices medicine. If I am a bad driver (traffic tickets and accidents) I will lose my license and/or pay much higher insurance premiums. Why not do that with physicians? Too easy. Too simple. Better to add to the patient's burden. So the wrong leg was removed. So you had a stroke because no one monitored your blood pressure. So you will be disabled for the rest of your life, cap the award because society can't expect physicians to pay more for insurance. Why not cap the premium insurance companies can charge physicians? No, that would be too simple. So make the patients pay for the wrongs done to them, which certainly is the American way. Those with the least power should always bear the burden.

One final event dealing with the lawyers and I will move on. They are not worth the time and space given the positive things I want to say about Susan's heroic effort to regain her dreams and live her life to the fullest.

There was a clause on the contract with the law firm that expenses and 10% of the settlement/verdict would be their payment. If we lost we were responsible for all expenses.

The doctor wanted to settle and become untangled in the potential trial with the hospital. I think he felt there was nothing to gain in arguing that everything went well. When he agreed to settle, the lawyers prepared a document for Susan to sign that, in part, read: "due to extraordinary effort in this case on your behalf our fee is now 20%." There was no trial, nothing out of the ordinary; the attorney for the physician brought up the issue of a settlement. Our attorneys were doing their job – what was the extraordinary effort? In fact, Susan had made the point of settling with the physician so that the case could concentrate on the hospital. It wasn't like we were off on vacation, not intimately involved in discussing this case. Nevertheless, Susan signed this amended agreement. I thought she should because what else do you do, change lawyers; hire a lawyer to review "your lawyer's" demand? Plus, our legal team is still preparing for trial against the hospital. So it was signed.

When the hospital settled, the lawyers wanted the 20% for their extraordinary work for the hospital as well. We said we never agreed to that. The lawyer said Susan did and produced the aforementioned letter. Susan said that the letter she signed had to do with the doctor. The lawyer responded, "The language says 'in this case.' The hospital is 'this case.'" That was never explained to us, and the law firm was happy to rip Susan off in the name of justice and their fee.

Susan's lead attorney told her, "If I was in your situation and could settle for a sizeable award to take care of my family, I would." Clearly this attorney was thinking of her payday. Perhaps, if this attorney was in a situation similar to Susan's, she would realize that no amount of money will give you your life back.

Finally, at the time the hospital was preparing for a settlement/trial with us, it was about to open and dedicate its new medical center complex. The hospital's PR theme was "Amazing Things Happen Here." Susan told her attorney that the hospital wanted to avoid all bad PR at any cost. Her attorney dismissed this suggestion until the hospital insisted on no publicity about Susan's case for 30 days after the opening. Clearly our attorney had no clue what was occurring – yet she felt compelled to request 20% for extraordinary work. Needless to say Susan was "very amazed" at what happened to her.

Sixteen years have passed and a new Prentice Women's Hospital has been built. Their PR campaign's tag line is "to be treated with respect and then, to be TREATED." Neither happened in Susan's case. The hospital and the physician abandoned her. No one cared. It was a blatant disregard of her medical needs.

Clearly, these attorneys and the way in which law is used to avoid responsibility are a sore point with me, Susan, and anyone interested in fairness and justice.

"True hope dwells on the possible, even when life seems to be a plot written by someone who wants to see how much adversity we can overcome. True hope responds to the real world, to real life; it is an active effort."

- Walter Anderson

June 17, 2004
Cleveland Clinic/Epilepsy Monitoring Unit

After almost twelve years fighting this battle against the consequences of a stroke and the relentless, unpredictable nature of epilepsy, we are in Cleveland. Conversations with neurologists and internet searches led us to the Cleveland Clinic. In truth, we have been to or talked with individuals at most major epilepsy centers. Cleveland, by default as well as by design, was next on the list. Besides, Susan's seizures were so out of control that we privately wondered if she could hold out until her scheduled appointment in Cleveland.

As we were driving to Cleveland, Susan asked me to promise – "Promise what?" I asked. "This is the last, the very last time I am going to go anywhere for any more EEG monitoring. This is the last dance. We have been everywhere there is, there is no where else to go. We have talked to practically everyone who is anyone, so this is it. No more." "Ok," I said. Stating the obvious, but knowing if there was a reason to do this again, a very good reason, I think Susan would do this monitoring again.

The only certainty over this span of time has been the paralysis from the stroke and the daily, never ending, devastating experience of epilepsy. Epilepsy is brutal. It is still here. Rampant as ever. Still trying to find anything that can help reduce and/or eliminate the seizures. More importantly, Susan is still battling. To say we are engaged in a fight to the death would not be overstating the situation.

Presently, Susan is hooked up to 25 or so scalp electrodes which will allow for the monitoring of her brain activity. This is the fourteenth time she has had EEG-video monitoring. She is sleeping, more accurately, she is so drugged from the medications given to break the status (status epilepticus is a state of repeated seizures that last for 30 minutes or longer; she has been in status for two days!) – that she cannot stay awake, even if she tried.

The seizure activity, while fairly constant at 2,000 or so seizures per month over the past few years has been exceptionally debilitating for more than three months. Seizures have a life of their own; they do as they please, while robbing Susan of any quality of life.

What is different about this round of seizures is both the increased frequency of seizures as well as their severity. When the seizures come in a particular pattern, it can be very troubling. That is where she is now. Susan has been "going left," her visual seizures are so strong that she turns to her left to "follow" the flashing lights or shooting stars or whatever the visual display might be. In addition, hallucinations occur, and present as people behind her, or with her, or she sees shapes/shadows dart across her field of vision. In her sick humor Susan jokes that when she is "certain" that I am next to her and behind her, she knows she is in trouble. "One of you is bad enough. When there are two of you, I know things are not right and it is time to be hospitalized." So going left and seeing people who are not present are indicators of a very serious cycle of seizures. While these events are occurring, the routine seizure activities continue: involuntary finger movement, toe movements, sharp pain, absent stare, all of which form a steady stream of seizure activities and their consequences. More medications are taken to try and interrupt this downward spiral of seizures. The medications add to the problem by increasing drowsiness, causing a sense of confusion/forgetfulness – an overall sense of being in a brain fog. Nothing is clear – except the persistence of the seizure activity.

Such constant seizing makes it difficult for Susan to walk, function, or really do anything. Postictal (the period after a seizure) headaches are almost incapacitating and the continuous nature of this brain unrest makes it very difficult to function, to be yourself to enjoy anything.

This state of affairs has been ongoing for more than three months. Thus, the effort to try and find out what could be done to help continues. We search for any new ideas, any hope, any way out. While we search, Susan hopes to be able to ride out this increased activity as if it is a storm. Often she will say, "If I can just get through this stretch, I'll be ok."

It is important to state that the struggle to find a cure or more specifically get answers and relief from the ongoing seizing is a very draining struggle. It is as difficult as anyone can imagine. The daily effort to undertake small tasks requires a personal fortitude that for many is not easily summoned. But Susan does so each and every day. Cheerfully, I might add. Nevertheless, the struggle is demanding and a heavy burden has to be confronted every waking moment of everyday. The fact that Susan has succeeded in fighting this battle for almost 12 years is virtually incomprehensible. Therefore, a statement which indicates this trip to Cleveland is "the end of the road" is all the more impressive in light of the burning question, "Why hasn't this ultimatum been made before?"

"End of the road" represents a momentary pause, a break to catch one's breath in preparation for the continuing struggle to beat epilepsy for herself and for others.

Susan's spirit is strong, her resolve unbending, her outlook is exceedingly positive. I, and those who come in contact with her, feel her energy and sense her willingness and determination to push on when others may have quit. She continues to fight. In spite of a 12-year battle, she is as fresh and ready to confront the day as if it was the first day in this journey. Her demeanor and disposition are truly remarkable.

Why Cleveland? Why now? Even though I start here, there is an epic story to relate between the end of the first few years and now. That will be told, but Cleveland, in many ways represents a turning point, a watershed that having been crossed, will not be considered again.

Over the course of time, the seizures have continued to increase in frequency and severity, and periods of continual seizure activity have been quite frequent. Best to think of the seizure total as a mountain range: the lowlands and foothills run on for a span of miles until higher elevations are reached before heading to the tops of the range. Susan's seizures resemble this pattern. A slow steady climb of the number of seizures: per day, per month, per quarter, per year, over years.

Whenever a plateau was reached it seemed like this period of time was a pause in the continual upward climb higher and higher.

When 20 to 30 seizures a month was the norm, it quickly was replaced by 20 to 30 a week, and over time to 20 to 30 per day – some days even higher.

In January, 2004 Susan's 1,200 to 1,400 seizures per month jumped to well over 2,400, practically doubling. There was no way to account for this increase. Susan could never identify any specific trigger or pattern of activities that correlated with the seizure pattern or frequency. As individuals with epilepsy know all too well – seizures have a mind of their own. Also there is a phrase "seizures beget seizures." It's as if once seizures start (and who knows why they start) they get on a roll until they stop (and who knows why they stop).

During a January 2004 hospitalization to monitor seizure activity and try and shut them down, the idea of another brain surgery was brought up, not for the first time, but this re-introduction of this surgical option was presented in quite dire terms.

"Perhaps you need to seriously (and the neurologist sounded very serious as he presented this idea) consider a right hemispherectomy." Susan tried to grasp these spoken words through the medication fog she was in. "Consider what?" she responded. "A right hemispherectomy or multi-lobe resection, maybe that sounds better to you." This is the same neurologist who initially raised this surgical option a year prior to this hospitalization.

I am not sure if the neurologist was trying to lighten the tone of the recommended surgery by offering a new phrase to describe it as if he was trying to be clever. I attempted to clarify things by blurting out, "You want to do another damn brain surgery to remove her brain, her right brain – is that right?" The neurologist replied, "Simply put, that is correct."

Simply put! Who is crazy? Removing half of a person's brain with the hope that the seizures will stop. Nothing is guaranteed about "curing" the seizures. But the phrase, "in the hope" stuck in my throat.

"You have to be kidding," I said in disbelief as I looked back and forth between the doctor and Susan. Directing my question to Susan, "He is kidding; he's nuts. What kind of suggestion is that?" Susan replied, "I don't think he is kidding, this is no joke."

Talk about an out-of-body experience. Here we have the neurologist, a colleague of his, a medical student, and Susan and I in her hospital room much like the outpatient visit a year ago when this option was first raised. And the idea they propose then is the same as now – to remove the right side of her brain.

The problem with this plan is that we have heard it before from them, from a neurologist at the Mayo Clinic after an extensive diagnostic assessment evaluation and then again from a neurosurgeon at UCLA. So, the idea being proposed was neither new nor a surprise. In fact, this very neurologist had suggested this surgical option at least twice before. Regardless, it was shocking. Shocking because of the tone in which it was presented. It did not seem like the surgery was an idea up for discussion. Rather, this is what is needed. You need to do it. End of discussion.

Ever since this idea of a right hemispherectomy came up in early 2003, it is the only thing we have been thinking about/considering. Now to have it put in your face as if time is up, next move is Susan's, is devastating.

"We'll have to think about it," Susan responded measurably. "I want to talk to the neurosurgeon and get a clearer picture of what is being proposed, the drawbacks and the benefits, the complications, recovery rates, and death rates." Can you imagine inquiring about the "death rates" from this procedure?

I was impressed by the calmness in Susan's voice. The deliberate way she responded to the proposed surgery was something to behold. I knew I would have been out of control or about to go out of control as I had already demonstrated by my initial reaction to this idea. Not Susan! She was calm and reasoned in her remarks. I thought to myself, excellent response. Take it under advisement and maybe the idea for more brain surgery will go away by itself. We can leave and we do not have to return. Let's just get out of here before anything bad happens.

As far back as the Spring of 2003 the seizures seemed to have moved to a new elevated level. That is not to say that the

252

period of time prior to this qualitative shift was ok; it was far from ok. The difference at this point in time was a significant increase in both the frequency, duration (length of seizure activity) and intensity of seizures.

Susan had sort of gone on a few mini-tours of neurology centers. She had met with doctors at Indiana University School of Medicine and at Rush Medical Center. She tried a consult at University of Chicago but that proved unproductive. Since epilepsy appeared to be gaining an upper hand she tried a consult at Mayo followed by an important evaluation session at Mayo.

Susan is, on occasion, asked to be a speaker at a medical conference or physician training program. When she presented at an epilepsy conference that had as its theme "Living Well With Epilepsy," a neurosurgeon was so moved by Susan's story that he sought her out and offered the option of sending film for him to review and comment upon. Without really knowing her, let alone examining her, his suggestion for the very surgery being proposed was consistent with the others, a right hemispherectomy – functional hemispherectomy was the way to go. But who in their right mind (excuse the pun) would go down this path? It is bad enough that some children have to endure this procedure. Such a procedure is rarely proposed as an adult treatment strategy. Yet, here it is being proposed to Susan.

The nightmare situation in the spring of 2004 became even more frightening. Seizures were now running at 3,000 per month and Susan was using additional medication to try and break this ever-rising cycle of seizures. More seizures, more drugs, more of her life being lost.

Between the non-stop seizing, increased dosage of her typical medications, plus the extra medication to try and break the cycle of seizing, it was extremely difficult for Susan to function at all. It was hard to wake up in the morning, let alone stay wake during the day. It was difficult for Susan to shower, dress and even make it to the kitchen table without feeling exhausted.

Walking was impeded; thinking impaired; and the ability to comprehend and process information compromised. It was seizure after seizure, take meds, get to bed for perhaps relief overnight (if the seizures didn't awake her during the night) and the cycle would repeat itself the next day. Day after day. Relentless.

As had been the case on countless occasions in the past, Susan would eventually say, "Somebody has to know what to do or where to go to figure out what can be done. There has to be something that can make a difference, somewhere." Thus, the stimulus to ramp up motivation and the hope machine and embark on trying to find answers and hope.

Susan's Ob/Gyn's husband is a neurologist who specializes in neuroanatomy and neuro-intensive care treatment. I sent him a detailed email as to what we were up against.

After reviewing records and gaining a sense of the current situation, he suggested that the Cleveland Clinic might be a place that could offer some information that might be helpful. That's all one needs. The slimmest of hope that there might be, could be, perhaps possible help somewhere and we were off and running. Whatever the word or phrase, any opportunity/new idea became the force for renewed efforts to find a cure/a solution for the seizures. To do nothing is to give in – surrender. Taking action reinvigorates hope. In the end, hope is all that is left.

A suggestion was made that the Cleveland Clinic would be worth a visit for an evaluation. Various web searches/email communications indicated a Dr. Najm would be the person to see. We made contact, sent information (x-rays, reports, labs, films, etc.) for his review and had a lengthy conversation with him about what an evaluation entailed. Susan felt it was worth the effort to try and bring closure/consensus as to what to do – what can be done, what options are open.

The week before the June 22, 2004 visit, Susan's seizures became particularly serious. Although she has multiple types of seizures, the ones that cause her to "look left," to see what is not there, experiencing hallucinations, and the almost continuous cycle of non-stop seizing indicates grave danger.

Susan decided to call the Cleveland Clinic to see if she could be admitted earlier than the scheduled evaluation. It was either an early admission to Cleveland or she would have to be hospitalized here in Chicago. Dr. Najm was able to arrange an earlier admission. We drove the six hours and experienced a few of these serious type seizures during the ride. I was extremely relieved to arrive in Cleveland. A brief side story to indicate the value-critical importance of humor. On the way to Cleveland, at a road stop rest area, we stopped for food and a bathroom break. Susan had gone to the rest room. Quite a bit of time had passed without her reappearing. I was about to ask someone who was going into the women's washroom to look for her when she appeared. "I was worried about you," I said, continuing, "I was about to go in and find you." "Have no fear, Bill," Susan exclaimed. "You were in the stall with me all the time; wherever I looked, you were there. I actually told you to leave and give me privacy when I realized you weren't really there." This made me feel supernatural to be able to be in two places at once. It also made me realize that it was important to get to Cleveland ASAP.

Susan saw Dr. Najm in the outpatient clinic. She was seizing throughout the appointment and after 45 minutes she was transported to the inpatient unit to be hooked up for the video EEG monitoring. From her perspective "let the Cleveland Clinic get a real good look at what I experience."

After a few hours of EEG video monitoring two things were clear: 1) the areas of seizing and the types of seizures were already well-documented and 2) she could not stop seizing in spite of efforts to stop them. In effect, the three day planned evaluation ended in a couple hours. Enough seizure monitoring data had been collected to document the nature and scope of the epilepsy. The challenge became slowing down the seizure activity and returning Susan to baseline. Stopping seizure activity all together is impossible – aside from a coma state, Susan always experienced seizures. The goal is to return to Susan's steady state prior to this eruption of seizure activity. Ever since the epilepsy surgeries in 1996, Susan has not been seizure-free. Not once over the past 3,650 days. Why the physicians at the Cleveland Clinic thought they had to totally stop the seizures is beyond me. Elimination of all seizures had never been accomplished by anyone or by any medical intervention. The goal was to return to the "normal" baseline of seizure activity without the extreme frequency and intensity that led us to the Cleveland Clinic in the first place.

This is why we are in Cleveland. While trying to stabilize Susan was the primary objective, the equally important goal of this visit was to obtain an opinion from the Cleveland Clinic as to what courses of action for addressing the epilepsy are available. What did they think? What options are available? What would they recommend?

By the end of the second day the seizures were continuing and physicians at the clinic had hoped to obtain additional test data, like an MRI and a neuropsych exam. I don't know what they were thinking, but Susan was in no shape to participate in these tests. Susan realized this and so did I. The fact that they didn't realize this made both of us wonder. I am amazed that these physicians at the Cleveland Clinic would even suggest such tests. Someone who is being bombarded by seizures, feels dazed due to the medications, and struggles to talk and/or stay wake certainly would not do well on the neuropsych testing, assuming she could stay awake during the test. The ongoing seizures prevented her from lying still. I'm not sure what an MRI would reveal under these circumstances. Besides, I had brought all of Susan's films with, so the need for another set of films and or another neuropsych battery seemed over the top. But all doctors want their own tests. Just adds costs. Nothing else.

Once these constraints on the testing were brought to their attention – multiple times, physicians at the clinic concurred with our position – no more testing was needed.

Susan, in spite of her condition, knew enough to tell the neurologist to give her a bolus – a maximum load of medications versus a few pills every few hours to try and shut down this excessive seizure activity. This was the only strategy that had worked in the past to try and break the seizure cycle. Overwhelm the brain to the point right before a coma and it might quiet things down. Eventually this suggestion by Susan was implemented and it ultimately succeeded. However, keep in mind that Susan is directing her care in order to break the seizure cycle. Cleveland had not figured this out. Where would Susan be without Susan?

By Friday afternoon we were scheduled to have a visit by the neurosurgeon and gain his opinion on the initial evaluation. The 5:00 p.m. afternoon visit arrived and so did an entourage of medical associates.

"So what do you think?" Susan asked the neurosurgeon or anyone else in ear shot who wished to venture an opinion. The surgeon, sort of an imposing figure not lacking in confidence (which I guess is a good thing if you are the surgeon and/or the patient) blurted out, "I'm recommending a functional right hemispherectomy. I would disconnect the right hemisphere from the rest of your brain and disconnect the lobes in the right hemisphere from each other, probably cut out some stuff as well. All of this," he continued, "should not cause you any more problems, because you are already paralyzed on the left side; your sight is impaired on the left, and you might not be able to walk, but that is it." That is it. Simple as that. And you might not walk – no big deal to him I am sure.

One of his technical remarks caught my attention: "probably cut out some stuff as well." I had expected a bit more medical terminology, the use of words that I could not pronounce or spell. But "stuff" was just too vague for me. "Might not walk" – easy for him to say. Maybe he should experience what it is like not to walk before dispassionately offering this result as if it was merely a minor inconvenience. Perhaps, if some of his "stuff" were to be removed he might have a different view of "stuff."

Susan said, "Really?" Nothing more, nothing less. As she sat in her bed with a pad of paper, pen in hand she continued, "I have a few questions I would like answered." She proceeded to rattle off four or five significant and profound questions: What are your results/success rates? How many adults, like me, have you done this surgery on? What are the complications and risks? How will I be after surgery compared to now? Will I have my mind, my executive capacity (i.e. higher-order thinking)?

For the most part, the neurosurgeon provided brief responses; very little elaboration, and what appeared to me to be sort of off-the-cuff guesses. "I have done 15-20 adults, all are seizure free (but he could not tell us what types of seizures they had). Counting children, we have a 70-80% success rate" (success was never defined). "You will be about the same" (what does that mean?).

Will she walk or not? Will she have cognitive deficits on top of what she experiences now? Fundamentally, will she still be Susan or not even remember who Susan was let alone our son?" Answers to these questions were not as forthcoming.

Despite on-going seizures and her drug impaired condition, Susan knew that it all didn't sound quite right. The icing on the cake came when the surgeon indicated he could do the surgery on Monday – three days away. The decision to buy a chair, table or any other household item requires us to shop around and think about it, but the decision to proceed with surgery should be made now! It didn't seem right, so Susan opted to become stabilized as best as possible and get the hell out of Cleveland.

As their brief encounter was ending, a colleague of the neurosurgeon offered the following comment directed at Susan: "Not having the surgery puts you at a higher risk than having the surgery." What "higher risk?" Death? Like being in a minimal cognitive state is a better situation! This doctor must be joking. Susan was clearly going to roll the dice. She had to think about what to do. Who to talk with. Despite being stunned, Susan knew enough not to proceed until she knew more.

Prior to leaving the hospital Susan decided that she would schedule the surgery, to "book it," just in case it had to be done and at the same time re-visit the neurosurgeon when she felt better, felt like herself, so that she could get straight answers and he can see how she really is when not in this drug-induced, "snowed" state of mind.

In between this discharge and the follow-up visit to Cleveland, Susan and I would explore all there is to know about this recommendation and what it actually meant; namely, what would be her likely cognitive state after such a surgery.

During the two weeks between visits with the neurosurgeon we tried to find out as much as we could about this proposed surgery. The more we learned about it, who is a candidate, and what outcomes can be expected, the less surgery became a viable consideration.

Clearly, it was rarely done on adults; it was mainly performed on children who already had profound cognitive problems. Unfortunately, the surgery leaves one side of the body paralyzed. To the families of these children, there are no easy choices. In Susan's case, she already had paralysis on her left side, but she could walk and had limited use of her left arm. Would this be lost? Susan needed answers not guesses.

We contacted other neurologists to obtain their opinion. One day an e-mail was received in response to our requests for an opinion regarding the surgery. The e-mail was quite long and detailed. The doctor read what we had forwarded to him and took his time in preparing a response. While not a vote for the surgery it was his comment that stunned us. "In sum, I strongly recommend against a clearly catastrophic and futile surgery that will leave you in a minimal state of cognitive functioning and with the likelihood of continued seizures." About as clear and devastating a response as anyone could write and one could read.

On July 1st, Susan called to cancel the July 7th surgery date.

The option of surgery, what it entailed, what it may mean to her cognitive and physical abilities, weighed on us like a ton of bricks. What else was there to think about? Shit has happened in the past and why not again.

Susan had discussions with her doctors at home and found comfort in the fact that they were very supportive of her decision not to proceed with the surgery. As one doctor said, "There are far too many unknowns to move ahead with surgery." Another doctor's comment went to the heart of the matter: "What is proposed goes to the essence of who you are. I am not sure who you would be after such a surgery, but I am confident you would not be who you are today."

Making this decision not to have the surgery was a great emotional relief to Susan. Nevertheless, she decided to keep the surgical consult/appointment with the neurosurgeon in Cleveland anyway. Susan wanted him to "see me as I am, not as some drug induced, almost comatose individual who can barely talk." The goal was to gain more information and to let the neurosurgeon see Susan and her capabilities. What would he say now?

As an aside, Susan was told that the neurosurgeon rarely does evaluations/consults like she has requested; he sees no value in doing it. He sees no value! I think a patient would value a leisurely, forthright assessment of what any surgery entails, let alone the type of brain surgery proposed. The good with the bad, especially the bad. What person would go forward with any surgery, let alone what is being proposed, without seeing and discussing the surgery with the surgeon <u>before</u> having the surgery itself?

We decided to fly to Cleveland on July 14th for an early afternoon appointment. The 16 hour round trip drive would have been too much to try in a day. We checked in at the outpatient clinic and awaited the appointment. We waited. No one is ever on time. Finally 45 minutes beyond the appointment time Susan's name was called and we were shown to a room to wait again.

The neurosurgical resident appeared, and said, "I'll review everything and answer all your questions before you see the doctor." The resident went over what was being proposed and didn't really add anything to what we had already learned on our own.

After this information session by the resident, he left and returned with the neurosurgeon. "So you are here to figure out what we are proposing and what you are going to do. How can I help?" he asked.

"I wanted you to know that I am pretty with it, unlike how I was when you saw me in the hospital two weeks ago," Susan said. "I can tell that," he replied. "Although, you were very aware of things despite all the meds you were on when I saw you in the hospital."

The neurosurgeon proceeded to explain the proposed surgery much like the resident had. Same pitch. Susan, having heard all of this before, waited until he was done and then said, "I have some questions I would like answered." "Fine, let's hear them," the doctor replied.

"How many patients, adults, have you performed this surgery on?"

"I have done about 100 or so; Cleveland has probably had the most experience with this type of surgery, and of those maybe three or five were adults. All were developmentally disabled and have had childhood problems that affected their brain development. They all did well and are seizure free."

"So cognitively I would feel the same? I'd be able to walk like I presently do? And more importantly, I could function at the cognitive level I currently do?" asked Susan.

"That's what I think. There really is nothing left on your right side (of the brain) but trouble which leads to seizures. I plan to disconnect the lobes from each other and from the left side of the brain and leave that disconnected tissue where it is. This should not be a problem," was the neurosurgeon's response.

"Can't the disconnected tissue shrink in volume which could lead to hydrocephalus? And when you disconnect the lobes, can't that be a new site for seizure activity?" To which he responded, "It could be." He continued, "but lots of things could happen and I don't see it being a problem." He added, "If you do the surgery you'll be here about three weeks and then return 2 weeks, 6 weeks, and 6

261

months after surgery so we can evaluate your recovery,
and then you are done. ”

As he was speaking I did not have a good feeling about the
surgery, especially since Susan is Susan except for the seizures. She
does not have the mental retardation that characterized the adult
patients he had preformed the surgeries on before. Could it be
Susan would be the first with such a clinical picture to undergo this
procedure? God help us.

After more small talk the surgeon said, *"I sense you are not*
really ready to commit to having 'the surgery'. ” *"No, I'm not ready to*
do this. I'm not sure if I'd ever be ready," said Susan. *"Let me ask you*
a personal question," Susan continued. *"If you were in my situation,*
or your wife, what would you recommend?" *"I'd do it, and I'd*
recommend my wife have it done as well," he responded.

"Thank you for your time; I now know what I needed to do.
Thanks again." As Susan finished her remarks we stood up and left.

We had a few hours to kill before going to the airport. We
found our way over to the cafeteria for a Coke. *"What a waste of*
time. Can you imagine he'd recommend that his wife have the surgery?
What an ass." My sentiments exactly. Susan continued, *"I have lost*
a lot of what I had or could do and I am not about to lose the rest. I'd
rather die knowing who I am than live and not know I'm alive."

We both heard the surgeon's answers to Susan's questions.
Later when discussing the appointment, we realized we had an
identical response to the neurosurgeon's observation "they all did
well and are seizure free." How could the other three or five adults
even know what was occurring, let alone be able to report on it
given their mental capabilities? All were severely mentally retarded.

The adults the neurosurgeon mentioned were mentally
retarded with significant cognitive and/or communicative deficits.
The surgery was done to address the seizures, but because they had
lost all there was to lose, their existing profound cognitive and
verbal deficits could not become any worse. In effect, the
neurosurgeon would not be in a position to know how well or
poorly the patients did post surgery.

So that was Cleveland. But it is the road to Cleveland that is a story in determination to find something or someone who could provide some direction as to what the course of treatment should be.

Another glimpse into health care will give you a perspective on the importance of not pre-judging a patient before one gets to know them.

Susan's doctor at the Rehabilitation Institute of Chicago (RIC) had not seen all the current work-ups, films, and reports. Dr. Smith, during this visit, took a long look at these documents and offered the following observation: "You know Susan, if I did not know you and who you are and only went off these films and reports to gain a sense of who you are, I would conclude that you probably can't walk, have significant cognitive impairment, and greatly diminished skills." "For me," she continued, "there isn't much more that could be lost if you proceed with the surgery."

Susan reflected and thought to herself, "I would have been written off and not seen for the potential I have. What a terrible injustice I and other patients are exposed to through such pre-judgment."

264

Chapter 11

SEARCHING

"To travel hopefully is a better thing than to have arrived."

— *Robert Louis Stevenson*

Searching. Looking for a needle in a haystack. Trying to find out who is doing what research aimed at curing epilepsy. You have to be committed and doggedly determined to find some treatment that could work because the epilepsy is not going to go away on its own. Searching, looking, will take effort and innovative thinking to "rethink" what to do about this illness.

Cure is the goal. Current approaches attempt to reduce seizures. Medications, surgeries and various implants are in the tool box of approaches, all of which have been considered, in light of the risks of these interventions vs. the hoped for gain.

Epilepsy really represents epilepsies – various forms, shapes, frequency of seizures, and consequences resulting from seizures. Such a range of clinical manifestations and resulting symptoms/difficulties present treatment challenges. There is a range of impairments and successful interventions that need to be developed to respond to the complicated set of epilepsies.

Susan's situation is unique in that she survived the stroke and the subsequent brain absess that eventually developed into intractable epilepsy. What is not unique is that from 35% to 60% (the number varies by study) of individuals with epilepsy do not have a treatment that works for them. The mantra "no seizures no side-effects" is a goal. It is not clear how many achieve this goal. Desperate things have to be tried when what is known to have worked fails.

An active chronic illness with varying episodes of acute flare-ups makes for a challenging life. Uncertainty is all that is certain. Susan believes, and I concur, that the relentless daily occurrences of seizures, and especially the all too frequent bouts of status, cannot be helpful for her brain. After 11 years, over 70,000 seizures, and all the anti-epilepsy drugs (AEDs) that have been taken, the cumulative insults cannot be positive for her brain or her overall health.

For example, try doing everything with just one hand, try it for a week; you may make it through a day. While you know this experiment will end, consider doing this "one hand experience" for 16 years, more than likely for the rest of your life. **THE** hand gets beat-up. There is "wear and tear" arthritis, carpel tunnel

syndrome, etc. Plus it is your **ONLY** hand. Lose the use of that
hand and you will lose – you don't want to think about what you
will lose.

Likewise, only one leg actually does the walking, weight
bearing. The left leg is barely functional. Somehow, through hard
work and practice, both of which continue daily, Susan was able to
re-learn how to stand and walk. Sixteen years of "walking" (we
joke that prior to the stroke we could never have considered how
Susan presently walks as walking) and she is able to hike up on her
right leg, swing the left leg through. But this adds wear and tear on
her right knee and even her hip. One does not have paralysis on
one side of their body and not have muscular consequences
everywhere.

For years Susan kept a log book in which she recorded her
seizures. It was helpful to count and plot the type of seizures and
examine trends or patterns. These seizure charts painted a picture
of the epilepsy far better than a phrase like "I have a lot of seizures,
not sure how many." In 2005, Susan decided to stop counting. The
only information she records are status events, extra anti-seizure
medications, ER visits, hospitalizations, "going left" and falls.

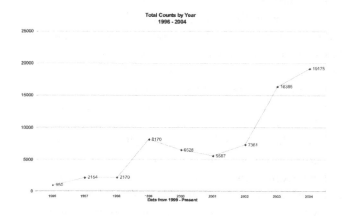

Looking at these data one can see the steady march
upward. In hindsight, after the 1996 epilepsy surgeries the
frequency of seizures at 40 or 50 a month seemed impossible to live

with. I recall thinking that having that many seizures would make it difficult for Susan to do the things she wished to do. What a misjudgment. There are days when Susan has 100 or more in one single day – or on many days in a row! Yet she still pushes forward.

Over a span of years the seizures escalated. More troubling was their increased intensity/severity. ER visits and hospitalizations were becoming frequent. It seemed like every three to six months some medical intervention was needed to stop the seizing.

New medications would be tried and/or the dose of phenobarbital would be increased. Susan was on a toxic level dosing of phenobarbital and the seizures would still rage. She takes Ativan, a drug to try and sedate, slow everything down, more frequently. One has to be extremely careful in using these drugs to slow seizures because these drugs can slow respiration and everything else. She doesn't need respiratory failure or a heart attack due to effort at stopping seizures.

ER and hospital visits, over time, occurred more frequently and present their own set of problems. Her veins roll and are difficult to penetrate as a result of the medications Susan had taken over the years. A problem which makes starting an IV or drawing blood extremely difficult. There is scar tissue from so many blood draws. Thus, starting an IV is a major task. In fact, more often than not when she is hospitalized, a central line has to be started because IVs are extremely difficult to start. When she is an outpatient, two to three "sticks" are common. More often than not, the blood draws are from her hand – sometimes her foot.

Over time it became clear that in emergency situations Susan needed a heavy loading of medication that practically put her in a coma so that the brain could be sedated, allowing for recovery from this electrical storm swirling in her head. The more medications she received the less she could remember and the more extended the period of recovery would be after each course of treatment. When she is "snowed" in order to stop the seizure activity, it can take up to 14 days to return to baseline – assuming no additional medications are used. The vicious cycle of meds to stop seizures stops her from truly living.

Clearly, this unrelenting assault of seizures on Susan's brain is a major concern. What a polite phrase: "major concern." Actually, I am very fearful for her life. These scare me (and I think her) to death. Nothing good or positive can occur as a result of this level of seizure activity. Nothing! It is potentially catastrophic. Can you imagine a heart patient experiencing this many palpitations or irregular heartbeats each day? Day after day. From my simple perspective, these seizures are further damaging Susan's brain. The seizures just pound away. The question we both have is how much pounding is too much and is there a point where the cumulative effect of this ongoing seizing will result in further cognitive deficits? Sort of a point of no return. In addition, all the seizure medications are not helpful to clear cognitive functioning. Taking 16-20 Advil each day for six years is also very worrisome, to put it mildly. We know about the GI consequences and potential liver damage that are monitored. But without the Advil, the headaches and arthritis would prevent her from living.

The potential for a steady decline in cognitive abilities "makes sense" to us; it has been suggested by the literature, and even her doctors begrudgingly acknowledge as much. The seizures continue unabated, which is why the search for a cure/treatment to reduce them continues as well.

One occasion in particular was such an alarming event that it pushed her to continue the search to find something, anything that would help. Our son has seen his Mom in very acute medical emergencies. He has seen her with wires coming out of her head; her shaven head – which revealed a labyrinth of scars from where her skull has been opened. Simply put, Matthew has seen things you wished he did not even know about, let alone witness. Such is our life and it is impossible to protect him or shield him from what occurs at home. He practically knows the paramedics by name due to their frequent visits to our home.

On this particular occasion, I was not at home. Matthew was seven years old at the time. While I was out at the grocery store, Susan had a major status event.

Status, uncontrolled seizing that lasts 30 minutes or more, is a life-threatening event. Typically there are no warnings that indicate a seizure or series of seizures will continue to escalate. This is precisely the problem; you don't know when a seizure will occur or what the course of the seizure activity will be. Susan sometimes engages in a form of the game "chicken." She has been through these events enough times that she is very willing to endure it without taking additional medications. She does so primarily on blind hope that the seizures will stop and because the added medications to slow the seizures will mean that she will "lose" the next seven days or more. It will be difficult to concentrate, she will be extremely tired, and she will fight to stay awake throughout the day. To avoid these negative experiences she is willing to chance that the seizures will run their natural course, whatever that is, and will eventually settle down on their own, thus avoiding the need to medicate or call the paramedics for an ER visit.

On this day, the constellation of troubling symptoms occurred rapidly. In "going left," seeing people and things that are not there, her left arm becomes rigid and begins to rise charting a course far above her head (normally she could not lift the arm very high at all, certainly not above her head). It is time for the extra medication. No need to wait to confirm the magnitude of this brain quake, at this point it may be too late to stop it at home and the 911 call is made.

Susan quickly realized that the initial seizure pattern was going south rapidly. All the signs of trouble, serious trouble were present and she asked Matthew to call 911 and get her the "special pills" she takes to try and shut this process down.

Matthew gave Susan her pills. Called 911 and described what was happening. He put our German Shepard in a bedroom so the dog would not be running around when the EMS people arrived. Matthew put the outside lights on and found Susan's medical summary sheet which is extremely helpful to the paramedics. He stayed on the phone explaining Susan's condition all the while trying to comfort her.

Once the paramedics arrived, Matthew even directed the paramedics on how to lift Susan since she is paralyzed on her left side and she could easily have shoulder damage if they weren't careful; he called me on my cell phone although I had seen the flashing lights up the street and knew what was occurring.

For his quick action in "saving his Mother's life" – as the citation reads, Matthew was recognized by the National Boy Scouts of America for his "cool under fire" and his "maturity in directing the paramedics as they assisted his Mother."

Matthew had been told what to do in case of an emergency. He knew where the medical information sheet was and where Susan kept the emergency medicine. But knowing what to do and actually being able to do it when such action had to be done are two different realities. Obviously Matthew is our hero. He did what he had to do in spite of the acute medical situation which had to frighten him.

I can only imagine what it must be like for Susan to "wait" 40 minutes to see if the seizures will break and slow down to a more normal frequency. Quite often there is only a short wait because the seizures escalate to a point where drugs administered under medical supervision has to be started. Oxygen is used to assist with Susan's breathing. The longer the seizures go, the more the respiratory system becomes compromised.

On another occasion, in a matter of minutes, Susan went from a normal day to status and even though a pill was tried there was no reason to believe things would slow down as a natural reaction to the additional medication. Susan had difficulty breathing. Her left arm was slowly rising above her head, like some Eastern exercise ritual, as her head and body slowly turned left, as if straining to see what was not there.

I called 911 as I slowly lowered her to the floor. She was becoming rigid and was about to slide off the kitchen chair. She lay on the floor shaking as if she was very chilled. Her head was turned left, staring at nothing, unable to look away and unable to speak.

It made me feel good to talk, so I did. "Keep breathing dear. I called 911 and they will be here quickly. Hang in there." The paramedics arrived quickly as though it never seems that way as you wait to hear the siren or see the flashing lights.

I gave the paramedics the one page medical summary which has anything and everything one would need to know. They tried to start an IV, but Susan's veins are scarred, hard, and they roll. After countless numbers of failed blood draws and IV attempts, they rushed her to the ER.

Well there was no luck and no skill tonight. The more they tried to start an IV the more time passed and even though she had oxygen her breathing was labored.

"Forget the IV and just get her the hell over to the hospital," I said to anyone who could hear it. "IVs are hard to start and we need to shut down the seizures. They have been non-stop for the last 50 – 60 minutes." The head paramedic acted on my suggestion.

In the ER, the nurse cut off her blouse and was close to starting a central line and placing Susan on a respirator. The goal was to stop seizures with a drug induced coma. Susan had received intra-muscular injections of some medication. The next thing I knew the blouse was cut off and the seizures appeared to be slowing. Susan had been "loaded-up" with enough seizure medication to put most people asleep for days. It was finally working. No respirator.

These status events generate a feeling of urgency to do something, which confronts a sense of despair in being unable to discover any intervention that would/could/might work. There must be someone who would know what to do, something that hasn't been tried, that could be tried. The eternal "there must be a care somewhere." Obviously we have searched and continue to search.

These increasing episodes of status alternating with hospitalizations started us on a track of trying to obtain a complete picture of just what is damaged, how extensive it is, how do the seizures propagate? These questions led to a decision to map her brain in order to evaluate options. Radiographic, EEG, computer-brain mapping, and visualizing seizures though dye markers, became ways in which both a complete and current sense of the brain damage could be made.

Major epilepsy centers around the country were contacted in the hopes of developing a diagnostic plan to address the intractable epilepsy. Our hope was that these efforts would yield a clear picture of what Susan's brain looked like, as well as what would be done. Two suggestions emerged. First, try the vagus nerve stimulator (VNS), an implant in the chest with wires up the left side of your neck that are wrapped around the vagus nerve. The implant sends electrical impulses to the brain on some sort of random bases in the hopes of dissipating the seizure activity. This had been a long standing recommendation.

Reviews on the utility of the VNS in Susan's case varied, but in general, there was little optimism for the procedure. As one neurosurgeon put it, "if you want to try it, I will do it and then in awhile I can remove it." The dismissal of the VNS was due to the extensive area of seizure activity, and we questioned whether an electrical stimulant could reach the deep areas of damage to do any good. In sum, could the electrical jolt get through the brain matter to dissipate the source of the seizures? No one knew. I had called the makers of VNS to discover if they knew of anyone with a history like Susan's that had tried the VNS. They knew of no one that would be comparable to Susan's set of circumstances.

The other suggestion, was raised in late 2002, and periodically after every difficult ER or hospitalization, since these medical interventions were all difficult, was more brain surgery.

At first Susan scoffed at the idea, a combination of disbelief and distain. After all, the last epilepsy surgery made matters worse not better. The neurologist who first offered this trial balloon suggestion characterized it as "disconnecting the right side of her brain." "Disconnect from what?" I asked. "From the 'left side,'" he said in a tone to indicate that my question didn't deserve an answer. And that's when I snapped. "So what is this supposed to accomplish?" His reply was, "It should reduce and maybe eliminate the seizures."

The word "should" did not seem right. Perhaps "it will" or "seizures will cease", something, some word that suggested knowledge rather than a guess or hoped for outcome.

"Do I even want to know the downside of this proposed surgery?" I asked. Susan interjected, "You are talking about doing a right-hemispherectomy, something done infrequently on children and rarely if ever done on an adult, especially a highly functioning adult."

"Would it sound better if I called the operation a multi-lobar resection?" The neurologist continued, "We could simply disconnect the lobes on the right side from the left side of the brain and from the lobes on the right side as well."

I was stunned that he was even suggesting this surgery. Susan remained calm and composed and merely said, "That's something to think about." Think about! Christ if the operation went ahead, Lord only knows if she would be able to think. Shit has happened before, a ton of it, and there is no reason to believe that shit can't keep happening. We are not immune from other life-altering events so why go looking at a surgery that could do just that?

This would not be the last time this surgical suggestion was raised by this doctor as well as others. While there is clearly the driving need to do something, there is no obligation to do or try something that can worsen the situation. As you can tell, I used the word can, not could or might. I'm concerned that nothing good could ever come from this proposed surgery – ever.

But the seed has been planted and the escalating seizures and life-threatening situations will foster its growth over the next several years. Susan's strategy to confront this suggestion was to realistically assess what could or could not be tried. Clearly, the hospitalizations and ER visits take a tremendous toll on her life. Days are lost due to the amount of medication administered; memory of the events over time is vague at best. What happened? The questions are endless because the void is great. There is a need to fill in the days with experiences. Yet each "I didn't know" or "I don't remember" reinforces how much of her life is passing by and she is unable to participate in it when there is a massive dosing of medication to stop the seemingly unstoppable seizures. The search to do something begins with a set of diagnostic procedures. "Brain mapping," overlapping EEG seizures within the structure of her

274

brain, was suggested. My guess is this test will show what areas of the brain are alive vs. dead; the dead being the areas of active seizing.

Taking the test is one thing, obtaining the results and the "so what" of the test is another. Susan waited for about a month for the appointment to review the brain mapping results. "Basically almost all of your right side of the brain (he touches her head over her right eye and touches her head behind her right ear) from the right temporal lobe back through the parietal lobe is useless. It is the source of your seizures. However, your seizures tend to dissipate over a wide area of the damage which accounts for the variety of seizures that you experience." The neurologist continued, "A bad brain is worse than no brain." I thought to myself, "What type of slogan is this?" So I added my version, "Just like your answer is worse than no answer." Not sure he got it, so I continued, "How do you know that all of the areas identified within the bad brain are bad? Maybe there are some neurons firing off which allows Susan to stand or walk or whatever. Are you totally sure of this?" "Well that is hard to say," the neurologist replied vaguely. That is just the point, I thought. Since no one knows, why is he or anyone else so sure of their suggestions? Maybe something is still viable on her right side that allows her to do certain things. If you disconnect the right from the left and all the lobes on the right from each other who knows what would happen? What would be left?

Fall 2003

Susan went through another procedure at Mayo Clinic in which a dye is injected right at the time of a seizure and a CAT scan is done as soon as possible which is supposed to visualize the damage. Ironically, while at the Mayo Clinic with video EEG monitoring occurring and seizures being captured on film, Susan receives an email request to speak at a conference entitled "Living Well with Epilepsy." Clearly the organizers do not have a clue about epilepsy. Susan accepted the invitation. I am eager to hear how she and others live well with epilepsy.

The evaluation at the Mayo Clinic stretched over a few days. A review of the information had to occur before any recommendations/suggestions could be made to her. Susan and I had to return to the Mayo Clinic for the presentation of the findings, following a department review of her case. Susan had meetings scheduled for a month after her discharge to return and talk with the neurologist and a neurosurgeon. Having appointments with both indicated to us that the idea of surgery would be raised again.

The neurologist indicated that a "right hemispherectomy" was the way to go, given the losses Susan already had and the likelihood that the surgery would not produce any additional losses of cognitive and/or physical functioning. I believe this was the third or fourth time Susan had heard this suggestion and the "it's not a big deal" pitch being made. The neurologist said, "I would rather refer to the surgery as a multi-lobe resection with extensive resectioning of the areas we feel are causing problems. There is no need for two surgeries, like you had before, the grid monitoring won't tell us anymore than we already know." So the plan would be one major surgery, which has enough risk in and of itself. Score 3-0 in favor of the right hemispherectomy. Obviously, Susan's vote will be the only vote that counts.

The next stop was the neurosurgeon. He was in the examining room as we walked in for the appointment. Our impression was that we would hear the same pitch for the surgery, so we were prepared for what was to come.

"My gosh, you can walk! I didn't know that. Wow, you can walk, this changes everything," the neurosurgeon proclaimed as we entered his office.

"What do you mean – I can walk?" asked Susan. "Who said I couldn't?" The neurosurgeon continued, "Well no one ever said you could walk; it never came up. I assumed from the films and reports about your brain damage that walking was not possible. This changes everything. I would have to have grid monitoring done to map your damaged area before we resected anything. So we are looking at two craniotomies over the course of three weeks. You can figure you will be staying up here about a month."

Reassured is not what I was feeling. Confident and competent are words that did not come to mind either. In a matter of 90 minutes, Susan received drastically different recommendations as to what physicians at the Mayo Clinic would do. These recommendations follow from the extensive case presentation/discussion with colleagues as to a course of action. Two surgeries are too risky as the neurologist sees things but absolutely essential as far as the neurosurgeon defines the situation. It made me relieved that we had sought out this consultation, what a joke! Keep in mind that at her case presentation to the senior faculty/staff no one had the thought to ask can she walk? This is a perfect example of how dismissive health care professionals or anyone for that matter can be. How many times are false assumptions made which markedly alter the course of care? In her case, the films and reports defined her – there was no need to see or ask her any questions.

During the consultation with the neurosurgeon, he noticed that Susan's left leg was swollen. Keep in mind we had just finished a six hour car ride. "Your leg is red, swollen, and warm to the touch. I would check it out when you get home. You may need an X-ray or something else. There may be a clot." Thank you for nothing. Raising the potential of a blood clot in her leg while allowing us to drive six hours back home did not seem prudent. "Keep your leg as elevated as you can until it is checked out," were his parting words to us. "Do you want to schedule the surgery now?" he asked. "I don't think I will. Thank you for your time." With that, Susan stood up and we walked out. "Let's head to the car and get out of here," she said.

This is and will always be the problem with searching—the extreme disappointment in failing to find a solution or resolution to the intractable epilepsy. What begins with determination and enthusiasm ends in disappointment and sadness. Every time we drove to Indianapolis to see Dr. Biller at the medical school we were positive and upbeat. The return home was always a let-down. The pain of these letdowns constrains your desire to "try again." Every failure ensures that the next effort has to have some plausibility of working or helping before Susan would subject herself to feelings of despair and hopelessness.

Returning from the Mayo Clinic, Susan decided she would "grin and bear it" – no surgery, nothing else seemed reasonable, so just put up with it. Even though the VNS did not seem plausible, its approach to activating the jolt of electricity to interrupt seizures offered an opportunity to explore. A watershed had been reached. Susan was seriously considering the VNS as a viable option. She first heard of it during the initial clinical trials of the implanted device years ago. After initially rejecting it outright, we are now so desperate that her physician is reluctantly "endorsing" it. The VNS was back on the table as an option.

Susan felt that the ability to activate the VNS as needed offered a tailoring of this electrical jolt. If the seizures got on a roll and she was in one of these prolonged cycle of seizing, could she activate the implant as needed, receiving 5 or 10 or 15 jolts, enough to penetrate the skull and deep inner brain region where the seizures seem to have their origin? Would rapid activation of the implant short circuit the seizing? At least that is how Susan phrased the question.

Reasonable question. Plausible result? Doing this repeated "wanning" to activate the implant, could that build up enough "force" so that it would disrupt the seizure activity? "I don't know" was the answer of the neurologist who had done the brain mapping. "I just don't know." I called the manufacturer of the VNS and no one could answer this question. I began to wonder if this is even possible. Could a "super jolt" be created by rapid repeated activation or does the effect of each jolt dissipate quickly?

Eventually, we reached our own conclusion; each charge sends out a single jolt. Repeated activation does nothing to strengthen the electrical discharge. There is no build up for a mega jolt. It is like having a life preserver on a rope; throw it out as far as it can go. It doesn't matter how often you throw it, it will only go so far.

In spite of a new openness to the VNS, the viability of this option as a way to address the rising seizure frequency ended quickly.

It is what it is and without options you simply go forward. There is nothing else you can do. While everything was pointing to a worsening of Susan's epilepsy there were pauses in the steady increase of seizures and medical interventions which simply allowed us to believe Susan had dodged a bullet. I think at some level we both realized this pseudo relief from having to decide what to do was time-limited. At any moment the march of seizures higher and higher could begin. If the seizures don't kill you, the uncertainty, unpredictableness of seizures will.

The fall and winter are busy times for us with Matthew at school and Susan's added responsibilities of getting him off in the morning, making lunch, keeping track of school events and homework assignments/projects. Susan gets up about 5:15 am to get ready, get the day going, and ride with him to school (Susan's dad drives them to school). School starts at 8:00 am, so Susan has already put in almost 3 hours by the time he is dropped off. Everything takes time, more and more time and one has to plan for this extra time for everything that needs to be done.

Winter 2003

While seizures ebb and flow, the direction has always been up and up in both count and severity. ER visits and hospitalizations were key events along this climb up. The winter of 2003 marked a beginning of an especially difficult period of seizing. "Going left," that is involuntarily turning her head markedly left as if to strain to see things around an illusionary corner or to catch a final glimpse of something before it quickly disappeared, is a sign of bad things to come. Add to this the experience of hallucinating, seeing people or things that are not present, also not a positive sign.

Susan is fond of saying that seeing me is scary enough, when she hallucinates and sees me both in front and back of her, or sometimes off to the side, that is too much to take.

Beginning about two weeks before Christmas of 2004, the seizures again noticeably increased, especially in their severity. There were more episodes of going left, more hallucinations, more episodes of simple status (seizing on or off every few minutes throughout the day), taking additional medications, taking more of the routine medication to try and stop the seizures. Whatever Susan could try to avoid being hospitalized at this time of the year she did. As the days passed, her ability to function markedly declined due to the combination of seizures, headaches, and medication side effects. It was difficult for her to remember what had to be done, if it had been done, or what things were put away (wrapped gifts, presents, etc.) . By Christmas Eve, she could barely stand but succeeded, somehow, to prepare the traditional Christmas meal, all the while negotiating with her physician when she could be admitted to the hospital to shut all this seizing down.

Family and friends arrived at 5:00 p.m. on Christmas Eve. Susan provided directions for my sister as to what to do, and we left at 5:30 p.m. for the hospital. I'm sure in her mind she beat the seizures. The seizures did not spoil Christmas Eve – but at what price? This is really not a game of winners/losers.

I am not always privy to Susan's mindset and what she is thinking. Can she really think things through when the seizures get this debilitating? Why not go in right away and stop them? "No, because I will be snowed when I leave the hospital." "Aren't you snowed while at home trying to do things while taking all the additional medications?" I asked. "Not as snowed as I could be," she responded.

Well she was right. Susan was admitted for little more than 24 hours (6:00 p.m. Christmas Eve through 4:00 p.m. Christmas Day). She had a central line started because an IV could not be started. An IV is the preferred route for administering medications. She had to be "loaded up" to such an extent that the use of a ventilator was being discussed because her breathing was being adversely affected.

Only because I explained how we could handle things at home and the fact that her routine doctor called to say it was ok for us to leave, did we leave when we did. Under different circumstances we would have been in the hospital for a week.

Susan's ability to stand unaided, walk without someone at her side, shower by herself, all were impossible following this hospitalization for almost a week. Remembering the events preceding the hospitalization, the hospitalization itself, the week after her hospitalization, as well as remembering that Christmas had occurred and what we did, who received what gifts, did Matthew enjoy himself, how did the Swedish meatballs turn out - was impossible. It is as if that period of time – even though she was participating in these events – is missing. It is gone like it never occurred, as if those events never happened. Experiences were lost unless I could help her recall them or she would ask specific questions which I answered. Even then, telling her what had occurred often didn't register. For example, Matthew and I visited Mom on Christmas day in the morning and he gave her two of the gifts he had for her. Susan did not remember the gifts (although she recalled the visit) even after significant prompting and discussing what took place. When she later found the gifts, Susan didn't realize that Matthew had given them to her or when she received them despite having gone over the sequence of these events numerous times. The drugs prevented events and experiences from registering.

This lack of connectedness to people, places and events, when explained as having occurred, presents a devastating reality to the person who has failed to remember experiencing them. Part of humanness is sharing, communicating, remembering; to miss these experiences is to miss living. It is to be present of body but absent of mind.

This particular hospitalization made Susan realize (she had already known this reality) that she was losing cognitive abilities and her physical functioning was declining. The seizures continued as expected following this hospitalization. Status had been broken. It took almost two months for her to feel like herself. She was left to confront the unknown, question when would it happen again, and whether it would it ever get to the point when extremely drastic measures might not work like they did this time.

Spring 2004

In May of 2004, the next time had arrived. Of course you never know this, either in advance or even while the seizures are escalating. You know only after the fact. The month of May, as the days passed, seemed to have more "bad days" than normal. It is not like "good and bad" days, it is more like typical days and days that are worse: excruciating headaches (which usually means ongoing seizing with some clinical manifestations) simple status (seizing throughout the day), more medications, going left, and occasionally seeing people who are not present.

Susan's Ob/Gyn happened to be married to a neurologist whose specialty was neuroanatomy and neurointensive care treatment. After a brief discussion with her Ob/Gyn as to what could possibly be done to address these unrelenting seizures, the idea emerged to contact her husband. "Tell him the story, tell him what had been tried, and see what he suggests." the OB/Gyn offered.

Susan's 50th birthday was approaching at the end of May and a surprise party had been planned. It could be cancelled if necessary, but I had high hopes it could be a wonderful party if all would go well. The universal hope: "if all would go well."

The doctor responded to our email. We also had an extended conversation by phone. The recommendation was to try the Cleveland Clinic, a place we knew of but had never thought of going to. However, having been to about every other place we decided to contact the neurologist he knew there to see what was possible. Sort of like trying to visit all the major national parks, might as well complete the neurology/epilepsy circuit.

The surprise 50th birthday party for Susan vs. the need to travel to Cleveland, which would occur first?

The cycle of turning left, seeing things that were not there, and the practically continuous pace of the seizures had returned, just like at Christmas. In five months she was back in the situation that usually necessitates hospitalization.

Fortunately the party won - a complete surprise. I had created a memory book which asked guests/family/friends to write down a most memorable moment they had experienced with Susan. The moment and a picture of the person who wrote it, were arranged in a memory book that Susan's niece created. A timely, lasting and meaningful gift.

Susan, unlike some who dread their 50th birthday, was thrilled. Living when, for all practical purposes, she should be dead, makes the celebration of this event truly special. Never expecting to see 50 makes getting here a tremendous accomplishment.

The joy of the day and the party were tempered by the upcoming visit that has been scheduled in Cleveland. The excitement of taking charge, taking action, to confront the epilepsy is a very powerful emotion. You're on the offense. However delusional it may be, you feel in control. While clearly that is not the case, you feel like it is. Something is being done that can maybe address the seizures. Maybe this time it would be different. Someone must know something, something that can be done. Maybe the Cleveland Clinic will be the place. Maybe.

Susan's birthday is May 22nd. Her appointment is for June 14th. As the days moved beyond her birthday, it was increasingly clear that it would be a miracle if she was able to last until the 14th of June. All the indications pointed to the need for medical care **NOW**.

Susan was routinely seizing throughout the day. More medication was being taken which only slightly diverted the onslaught of seizures. Seizing and taking medications were all that she could do. It had reached a point when she acknowledged what has been obvious but unspoken. "I'm either going to go to the Cleveland Clinic now or I will just go to Loyola and get snowed. I am beyond my limit to tolerate this. I have to go somewhere."

I called the Cleveland Clinic and explained the situation. "Come in tomorrow, we can see Susan and will have a bed available." Susan was relieved that something was going to happen. I suggested we go to bed early that night (seizures usually do not wake her up, or they can—another uncertainty) because it was an eight hour car ride the next day.

The Cleveland Clinic had an excellent reputation in epilepsy and other medical problems as well. While that reputation was a comfort it really didn't mean that much. What could they do for her? Susan's case was unique, tremendous brain damage, intractable epilepsy that is resistant to surgery and/or medications, yet high functioning and the ability to walk. Susan is a case that no one ever sees so the approach to treatment has to be outside the box.

Hopes, as always, are high when a decision is reached to take action aimed at stopping the seizures. Such was the case with the Cleveland trip. Collect the x-rays, reports, charts, medical records, test results, everything and head off. High anticipation and high anxiety! Great worry, however, is never far away. As we feared, Cleveland wasn't the answer.

We returned from Cleveland to Chicago late on a Saturday. Susan tolerated the trip, on and off sleeping and napping characterized the return ride. Exhausted, snowed, relieved that she had avoided the proposed surgery. We were both mentally and physically exhausted. We returned in time to attend an epilepsy fundraising event the following Monday. Susan and Matthew had participated in a photo shoot that was to be included in a video to be shown at this event. Friends were going to attend the fundraiser as well as Matthew. So it was important, very important, that in spite of how she felt it was imperative that we as a family attend this event.

Susan felt sick at the mere thought, let alone discussion, of this proposed right hemispherectomy surgery. During the presentation of the video, there were six brief case histories. In one, a mother talked about how devastating epilepsy had been and still was to her daughter. At age 16, the child's seizures were so out of control that the mother opted for the right hemispherectomy surgery, the one suggested for Susan. The mother recounted her painful decision. "It's your worse nightmare. Having to decide to allow the surgery to be done on your child, knowing that she will lose the use of her left side of the body, in the hope that the surgery will eliminate the seizures."

She continued, "So I said go ahead, and Julie was seizure free for about a month or two before the seizures returned. The doctor says she is having seizures not only in front of but also behind the area where they removed her brain. Nothing was gained and so much was lost."

I had a hard time breathing having heard "in front of and behind where they removed the brain." I looked at Susan and we both knew what the other was thinking, "What a difficult decision, for what? A nightmare, that is all it is: a nightmare!" Now Julie has uncontrolled epilepsy, and she is paralyzed on her right side.

Susan leaned over to whisper, "No way. I may be out of it and appear stupid to them given all the medications they gave me, but I am not going to do the surgery. I would rather die. At least I would be dead rather than being alive and having no realization that I am living. No way! No way! Never. It was meant that we see this. I should get a copy of this video and send it to the crew at the Cleveland Clinic."

If there ever needed to be a final nail in the coffin, this short video clip was it. The pain on this mother's face over the choice she made and the consequences of that choice are still with her seven years after the surgery. No doubt they are with her every time she looks at her daughter. I went looking for Julie's mother among the crowd at this event. After a while, I found her and introduced myself, briefly told her about the Cleveland Clinic, and identified Susan in the video. "For what it's worth, I hope you are at peace with the decision you made about the surgery for your daughter. You did what any parent would have done – try and give your child a better life. You need to believe that." She looked at me and said, "Thank you for your kind words."

That is how desperate people are to regain, or claim for the first time in a long time, their mind from the assault of epilepsy. To somehow remove the fog of medication; to think clearly like a sunny blue sky day; to feel unburdened by the side effects of medications that are supposed to help you, but which, in part, numb you to the reality of seizing. In some ways perhaps that is their purpose, their "benefit"- numb the person to the seizure experience. Whatever could do that, at whatever the price, may be worth it. Ask Susan and you will receive an unequivocal answer – NO! Anything that robs one of his or her mind – who one is – is not worth it.

Chapter 12
REFLECTIONS

"The past is only good if it helps you move forward."

- William J. Filstead

It is difficult to reflect on both the major and subtle events that have happened over these 16 years. All of these events have challenged us. Because of the disability and her need for assistance, in many ways, her life became my life. The delicate balance between helping and taking over; between asking vs. doing, between deciding what to do rather than discussing what should be done, the list is endless. This "what should I do" dance continues today and it will in all probability continue throughout our lives. It just is.

The challenge for Susan, perhaps more so for me, is to realize that whatever the future holds "it is her life," and no one should try and live it for her. I know she keenly realizes this. The struggle is for others to allow her an opportunity to control her life. Do not interfere. Provide help when asked. Do not impose help that is not wanted.

When a loved one has both a physical and cognitive deficit, the other spouse (at least I did) begins to think and act on their behalf. The key to maintaining a relationship or marriage after such a catastrophic event is to figure out, by trial and error, how things will have to be done to the satisfaction of all parties. It also should be said, even though it may seem like stating the obvious, if the relationship or marriage was in trouble or not going well before such a life altering experience, such an experience is not going to help maintain the marriage.

I have been accused of hovering, having an overbearing presence. There is a difference between being there and being in one's face. I had to learn, and since I am a slow learner, I am still learning 16 years later, what is needed vs. not wanted; what is helpful vs. hurtful; what fostered independence and does not create dependence. Susan was threatening to buy me a skull cap with a pin wheel on top so I could hover more efficiently.

Ask! Ask! That is where everything starts in a relationship. Ask before doing is a very good rule. It applies almost all the time and in all settings.

While it has been more than sixteen years since the initial stroke, our memory of our lives before the event is still fresh: what we did, what we liked and what our plans were. Every task or action taken because of the disability is a reminder of what we had, what she lost, and what is now different.

If my wife is in the bathroom too long, I will go by the door and ask, "Are you ok?" Never would I have done that before, but seizures have a way of occurring when they want to. So the question, "Are you ok?" is a way of checking to make sure Susan is not in trouble.

Susan has a "lifeline device," a pendant she wears around her neck. If she is in need of help she can press the button which dials a phone number to the local hospital. In a matter of seconds a voice comes over the speaker unit and asks, "Are you ok, Mrs. Filstead? Do you need help?" I never leave the house unless she has the pendant on. In fact, even when I am in the house she often wears the device.

When we are together, in the same room, I have my radar on so that I am alert to what might be going wrong. If I don't hear noise in the kitchen, I will call her name. Sometimes I hear her take a very deep breath which tells me she is having a seizure. I am always ready with a chair so she can sit down until the seizure passes. I am always ready; alert; watchful; ready to respond.

If Susan has a seizure while sitting and attempts to walk afterwards (Susan has difficulty with standing, her balance, and walking right after a seizure), I try to be there to offer a steady hand. She has to stand and weight bear to regain her capacity to walk. As soon as she stands, I stand and offer her my arm as a way to balance herself.

These examples of being aware occur almost automatically. I am alert to these situations and needs, and I choose to be always vigilant.

Anger – what can I say? Anger is front and center. Any situation or experience is an opportunity for anger to ignite. In fact, I don't think either of us could respond any other way. We acknowledge that such anger is not helpful or healthy—but at this point, there does not seem to be anything that either of us can do about it.

For example, today Susan was trying to put on her earrings, a special set which she rarely wears. She was having a hard time getting them in.

"Need help?" I asked.

"No, I need two hands! It is hard to get them in with just one hand," Susan bellows.

"I'll help you if you want. I can help put them in," I calmly reply.

"No! I would rather not wear them. I will just give them away since I can't use them anymore," Susan cries.

"How happy are you?" I ask sarcastically. "If you don't want them, maybe I can wear them?"

"That is just the point. There was nothing in particular bothering me and then all of a sudden I am over the edge. I get angry all over again. Angry at the hospital, the lawyers, and my life; add anything else you would like." The anger is palpable. "By the way, your face is too heavy for these earrings to work for you," Susan remarks.

This is an example of how any event can be the source of a major blowup and eventually a review (could be short or long) of all the things that went wrong. Then just as quickly there is the joke, the laugh that tries to defuse the situation, to help us forget the pain.

The seizures are a constant reminder to both of us about what didn't happen and how life could be if appropriate treatment interventions would have been made. In all likelihood, if Susan's vital signs were monitored and she received the appropriate care, I would not be telling this story.

We both know the anger, or should I say rage, we feel at times is not healthy. "You have to deal with it," says a psychologist. "You need to get on with your life," says someone else. Hurray for them!

Often our conversations will focus on why the anger. There are a great many people who experience heartbreak because someone they loved died, was killed, or suffered a horrific injury. While there has yet to be any conclusive resolution of the question, "Why the anger?" Susan has an answer that seems plausible.

> *"It really is quite simple. I have thought about this matter (the anger) for sometime. I never saw myself as an angry person so these feelings upset me. Why the anger? No one has taken any responsibility for what happened to me. No one has said I am sorry, or we tried (which they obviously didn't do). No one! Even the settlement stated that the hospital and doctor by settling do not admit guilt with regard to the charges. So no one has stepped up to the plate and accepted responsibility." She continues, "Add to this their efforts to lie and avoid responsibility. Dr. Toig even suggested a distant relative of mine had gout which might have contributed to my problem. How pathetic. The nurse, Lori, lied when asked about the decision to stay with me all day. The missing blood pressure chart that was found and obviously changed, need I go on? Forgive? I can't see it happening. Maybe if someone asked for forgiveness then the situation would be different. How can you forgive someone who believes they did nothing wrong? Are we to feel better by saying "You're forgiven?" That is not likely to work."*

As a point of clarification, Susan and I do not walk around all day, each and every day, in a rage. Far from it. Nevertheless, the anger is always present in some manner or form and asserts itself in response to a painful event, memory, experience or loss. It just does and I can't imagine it any other way.

Susan started a foundation, The Susan Eik Filstead Stroke and Epilepsy Foundation, Inc. www.SEFSEF.org, as a way to channel her energies and interests in finding a cure for epilepsy and the reversal of damage caused by a stroke. All too often success is measured by the criteria of seizure reduction and/or elimination of seizures all together. Achieving this goal may require surgery and/or medications, even multiple medications, sort of a heavy price to pay for seizure relief.

"No seizures, no side-effects" is the goal she strives for, both for herself and for others. Research has slowly gravitated to this perspective and to the issue of the patient's quality of life. Reducing seizures from ten to five a day is "an improvement," but if the medications taken to achieve this prevents the individual from realizing what day it is, what's the point?

It is worth noting that epilepsy has many manifestations and permutations. Everyone is not alike. The challenge is to find out what might work for whom to control or eliminate the seizures and the price to be paid to achieve this goal.

Research indicates three million individuals in the US have epilepsy. About 300,000 new cases each year from a variety of sources/injuries. Most people with epilepsy, if not all, take seizure medications, some more than one. About 35 – 40% have intractable epilepsy, that is, epilepsy that is resistant to treatment. All who take medication typically experience some side effects, the type of side effects, the degree and frequency of occurrence varying widely. Seizure medication typically leaves one feeling tired, perhaps not as mentally sharp, with slowed thinking and reaction to experiences. A fog or "low clouds," a dulled sense of things, also characterizes how one feels when on these medications. I would surmise that these experiences add to the burden of the seizures themselves. What one is, how one is reacted to by others, how one reacts, shapes one's sense of self. Who you are cannot just be seen. Who you are has to be experienced by others. What you do goes farther than talk about doing something.

People who have epilepsy often hide the side effects of the medications or the epilepsy itself from others, especially people who do not know them. Why would one want to expose oneself to the cultural and social stereotypes that surround this disease? After all, it is less than 100 years ago when people who had epilepsy were institutionalized in this country. People were believed to be possessed by the devil.

Susan has retained her executive function capacity and other mental faculties despite this catastrophic assault on her brain. If you saw Susan sitting at a table, you would not surmise that anything was medically/physically wrong. Her speech is clear, her conversation flows just like anyone else's. But during a seizure, she might stop talking mid-sentence. She may stare without seeing anything or connecting with anyone. She may have a debilitating headache due to the on-going seizing and the postictal period after a seizure. She may fail to remember what was being discussed or what was decided in the minutes before the seizure(s). One just never knows what the next moment will bring.

For example, I will tell Susan I am going to the cleaners in the course of small talk; she will have a seizure and when I say I am going now, she will ask "where?" I will say "the cleaners" and she will say OK as if that is the first time she has heard of this plan.

Trying to do more than one thing at a time is practically impossible. When a question is asked of her, and she is doing something like looking at her calendar or talking on the phone, there is usually no response to the question. Tasks, questions, etc. have to get in line and wait their turn if they wish to get done or be answered.

Creating structure, routine, predictability to daily activities has been a chief way Susan is able to accomplish as much as she can. Clothes are selected and laid out the night before, because it would be too much to do and think about along with showering the next morning.

All phone calls are logged on a daily calendar. All appointments and things to do are entered in a date book. Yellow post-it notes are everywhere. Granted many people do similar things, but in Susan's case it is both her style – she likes to be organized – and it is essential for keeping track of what has to get done.

The reality of who Susan is vs. who Susan was relates only to physical attributes. She is still Susan, the woman I married and love today. Assistance is needed for different tasks, some activities of daily living, or projects. For 16 years one hand has done the work of two, and the wear and tear is obvious. Arthritis in her hand, knees, and neck add to her declining physical state. She is upbeat, hopeful, and that is a miracle in itself.

Mr. No Man. That became my unofficial nick-name soon after the stroke. It seemed everyone wanted to do something or have something to do and the question was put to me often, "What can I do? Do you need help?" I would always respond, "No. We are ok."

To me trying to coordinate "helpers" was more difficult than doing it myself. My sister said she would wash the clothes, once a week. I would rather throw in a load or two at night and be done with it. Grocery shopping. I had no idea what I bought at the store (brand name, size, etc) so it was easier to pack-up Matthew when he awoke in the early morning and shop myself rather than try and construct a list.

There was help and I was very grateful for it. Our house was cleaned on a Saturday while I visited Susan. Various family members would watch Matthew or have him stay overnight so I could visit Susan later in the evening or get an un-interrupted night's sleep once in awhile.

I may have said this earlier in the book; but, the word stroke came to mind immediately when I heard the phone message to call the hospital. After all, Susan's blood pressure had been the issue throughout her pregnancy and especially the delivery. Silly me, I felt reassured (talk about a false sense of security) that Susan was returning to the high risk monitoring unit. What better place to receive care if care was needed.

I remember my mind racing as I drove to downtown Chicago, asking the receptionist, upon arriving, "Where is the stroke unit?" only to be told "This is the Women's Hospital".

I could not completely comprehend Dr. Biller's explanation of what had occurred until he said, "Your wife has suffered a catastrophic stroke, and she is paralyzed on her left side and cannot see out of her left eye. Approach her from the right and be strong for her. She needs you to be strong."

I certainly didn't feel strong or even capable of being strong, but when there are no choices one either does what has to be done or they don't. It is that simple. Very simple. I will always remember her first words to me, "Happy birthday Bill. Can you believe this?" Actually, her response was the best present I could ever receive. She had it together and, in spite of the dire circumstances, she cracked a joke.

A joke. Laughter. Black humor. Without these expressions. along with good natured kidding, we would never, ever, have made it. It is what allowed us to stop from going over the edge, or if we do go over the edge occasionally, humor pulls us back.

Humor blunts the pain. It makes the unbearable-bearable. For that exact moment laughter allows one to discharge fears, anxiety, anger, maybe for only the moment. But that moment is essential to regaining our composure and perspective. It allows us to catch our wind, pause long enough to resume the struggle refreshed.

I know readers might wonder how we found humor. What is there to laugh about? Everyday life is full of opportunities to laugh and fortunately Susan and I take every opportunity to do so. I recall a "Far-Side" cartoon that became her favorite. A man in a wheelchair said to a man standing "I'm not worried. Lightening never strikes twice, does it?" as a large bolt of lightening and a meteorite are about to strike him.

The days immediately after the stroke ran together. I recall being calm during this period. Perhaps I was in shock and could not comprehend the seemingly incomprehensible. What the hell happened changed our lives forever! I'm not sure anyone can grasp what that means.

Most people, I think, take their health for granted. After all, if you are not sick I am not sure you are rejoicing in your good health. Becoming sick, life and death issues, force you to look at your health. Health takes on an entirely new meaning. Illness is incomprehensible while healthy.

Living not dying was the first goal. Dying was a distinct possibility, a likely reality unless emergency brain surgery was done. Done sooner rather than later. Having lived, the goal became survival. Susan needed to recover, she needed to make it, not just survive the operation.

All efforts became focused on getting better and getting back to who she was. At the time we did not know that getting back to who she was would never happen.

All I knew and all I wanted Susan to know was "'til the end of time." We would be together no matter what. So the goal was to make us be a family. With Matthew in ICU for 2 weeks and Susan in the hospital for however long, the objective was to make us be a family.

With hindsight, I am not sure how things got done or how we kept moving along. You are in the river and the current is taking you for a ride. Days became weeks, weeks became months and we persevered. Once home, home care, nursing, OT/PT, others provided a constant flow of traffic. Life is a flow of experiences and we were in for the ride.

I honestly can't remember how we made it through the first year with the baby, work, multiple doctor/hospital visits, etc. It soon became clear: you did what you could. The rest had to get in line.

I do not ever recall feeling "sorry" for "all that I had to do," as my mother and my mother-in-law would often say. I complain a great deal in this book about having no time. Being overwhelmed. But the complaining was done to myself. I talked to myself quite a bit. Rarely did I discuss these frustrations with others. Susan heard my complaints more than anyone, and for that I apologize. I did what Susan would have done. A routine was established, and that helped structure all that needed to be done. I recall complaining to myself about the lack of time. Never enough time. A few years ago I stopped wearing a watch so I don't even know what time it is anymore.

The word caregiver is used almost universally to identity a family member who helps another family member because of a disability or chronic illness. I have never liked the word; I am not sure what word would be better. The point to note is that I helped as needed, the need determined by Susan. I am good at running the railroad. So my preference is to do everything, eliminate the guess work and simply take over. A big mistake. Susan has helped me learn this lesson.

Susan had to decide what help she needed and when. My role was to help out when asked, that's key, when asked. Time was no longer an issue. If I could do something in 5-10 minutes and it would take Susan 20 -30 minutes, then 20-30 minutes it was. That is not to say that there weren't many times when I just wanted to do it so we could get on with something else. I had to learn the value to asking if help was needed and wanted, otherwise, I would continue to rob Susan of the ability to accomplish what she could do by herself.

I can recall only one time when I felt we (I) had reached rock bottom. Matthew was in his terrible 2's or 3's or 4's – or whatever. I am not nearly as psychologically attuned as Susan and did not appreciate Matthew's anxiety and concern over being left at the craft program in the park across from our house. He wanted to go, but when we arrived, he didn't want to stay. We left to go back home and he cried because he wanted to participate in the craft. So we headed back to the field house, and the cycle repeated itself.

Eventually, we headed home. I decided that no matter what he said, he was not going to attend the craft program that day. Arriving home Susan greets us and experiences Matthew crying and me ranting something to the effect of, "This is it. I am over the edge. I have reached my limits." Since I had left his jacket at the park house, I turned to go back and retrieve it, still ranting.

While walking the 100 yards or so I felt death was a better option then life at that moment. "I don't give a shit if I die, at least I would be dead and someone else could help out." I clearly remember wishing to die; die now so I didn't have to walk back home. I went over to a park bench and began to cry uncontrollably. I am not sure why or about what. But I don't ever recall crying like that in my life, before or since that day.

Some time passed, I am not sure how long I sat there. I looked up to see the instructor approaching me with Matthew's jacket. "You forgot his jacket. I hope to see Matthew next time." "Yeah, sure. We will be here next time," I replied.

Upon returning home, I looked at Susan and said, "Perhaps I need to lighten up." "That is very insightful Bill. I am impressed," Susan replied. With that I gave her a kiss, showed Matthew his jacket and said, "Maybe Mommy can go with us and stay at the class with you next time, ok?" "Ok," Matthew nodded as he continued to play.

I felt very guilty about wishing to die, like I had it so bad. I have never felt that way since, and never wish to feel that way again.

Chapter 13
ANYTHING LEARNED?

"While there's life, there's hope."

- Marcus Tullius Cicero

I am not sure if we, speaking for myself, I – have learned anything from this experience. I am sure if someone had asked me hypothetically whether I could deal with such a situation I would have said, "I'm not sure." Privately, I am not sure I could have. No one really knows what he/she would do until it comes time to do it. That's the ultimate test. Put up or shut up.

So speculation about what would or could happen was quickly replaced with reality. You either do or you don't. One finds out quickly whether he/she can deal with the situation, whatever that means. In fact, it is ridiculous to even consider the hypothetical. Who has choices over such matters? It is not like there is a list of good or bad experiences and you can select what will happen. What happens - happens.

What we had going for us was that we truly loved one another; the "other" was the most important person in our lives. The "us" mentally makes us one. Did we expect such an event? No! Would you? Were we prepared for such an event? No! I believe we had wills, or if we didn't, I knew that we had to have wills quickly. Then again, beside the house and life insurance (not even sure what we had) there were no assets.

I am impressed with Susan and her determination and hope for the future. She demonstrates courage, drive, resolve, guts, each day as she deals with the results of the stroke and the on-going seizures.

She is not looking for help; she is looking for a cure. For herself, that would be nice, but also a cure so that others and especially children do not have to experience seizures.

Susan meets each day head-on. Despite the relentless seizures and the almost constant headaches which follow the daily round of seizures, nothing stops her. Nothing, nothing comes easy, yet the situation is what it is and she moves on.

Susan is soft spoken, but can command an audience. All attention is on her when she tells her story. The drive that pushes her was, and is, Matthew. To be there for him and to help him adjust to life. Susan established a foundation (www.SEFSEF.org) to increase public awareness of epilepsy and the signs of a stroke. Most importantly to find a cure. The foundation has given her a mission to help others in whatever way she can. That it has given others hope is exactly what Susan is about. Spread the word – hope.

While she isn't, as she says, the "Mom I thought I would be," Susan is Matthew's Mom and does whatever she can for him. Life is bittersweet. You tend to view events in some kind of flow or context. Either the past experiences or one's future hopes bracket daily living. But each experience comes with some baggage. We remember what we did when we were in San Francisco before the stroke in contrast to what we do now.

Loss, in spite of the gains and strides Susan has made, is always present. Sometimes it looms larger and more painful than other experiences, but it is always present. Life can be truly difficult. If you can acknowledge that fact, it no longer matters, life is what it is and especially what we make it be.

Susan was a "room mother" at Matthew's school, but I had to drive her, carry the food and supplies and help her set up. Not how she had imagined it, but the end result was that the kids saw Susan in the room as the room mom. That is what is important. Matthew can go on an overnight field trip to the museum with his friends in scouts. Susan can't go. It would be extremely difficult. I can go, but someone will have to stay with Susan should I stay overnight. Not the way we thought this would be.

While I will be politically correct and say I think of Susan all the time, I never planned to be thinking about how she is doing. How were the seizures? Does she have her lifeline necklace on? Who is with her? Never in my wildest dreams did I think these would be my thoughts of my wife.

Susan, as she often points out, would like to be left alone. There are times she would appreciate being alone. She wants to be by herself to do what she wants. She wants to have quiet, be capable of being alone, and have some sense of independence. Once Matthew and I were going somewhere and Susan was to be by herself for four or five hours. Of course, I felt someone should stay with her, but she insisted that she was a "big girl" and would be ok. "Besides, that is why we have the lifeline necklace. If there is any trouble I will hit the button and help will come." I reluctantly agreed to leave with Matthew. As I was pulling out of the driveway I called her from my cell phone. "Miss us yet?" I asked. "Sure do. Hurry home," she said. "I take that to mean we should stay away for a long while?" "Longer if you can!" she responded. And so it goes. At home I am watching, monitoring. When I am gone I worry. Should she go out with a friend I worry as well. Can she get into the car? Are there steps she has to walk down? Is somebody in front of her as she walks down the stairs in case she has a seizure and falls? Obviously, I am relieved when she returns.

I habitually use the word "we" when scheduling an appointment or "we" need to figure out what to do next. We, not Susan or me, but we. I am aware of this and at one level I do not like what the pronoun represents.

We (Susan and I) are unique individuals with distinct styles yet at the same time we (Susan and I) are the same as in" "we" need to figure out what the next step is? We are in this together. The stroke and epilepsy have modified our roles, responsibilities, abilities and our sense of self. On a personal level, each of us has been affected in markedly different ways. So collectively, we have been joined together as one in the response to this event.

Clearly, I have learned practicality. Life does indeed present challenges. Faced with a life-altering event, one responds rather than thinks about it. No time for reflecting.

Perhaps this assessment is too simplistic; perhaps there are more complicated explanations. There was a famous American sociologist in the 1920s who coined the concept: definition of the situation. Simply stated: However one defined a situation it is real in its consequences. So, if life gives you lemons you can be sour about life or you can seize the opportunity and make lemonade.

Laughter has saved us. It has made life easier, lighter, and more grounded in the flow of events rather than the ever present worry over seizures.

Earlier on, right after the stroke, family and friends tried to be comforting with their comments/remarks. A rule to remember; if you don't know what to say it is best to say nothing. Saying nothing is preferable to sounding like an ass. In spite of this universal truism, it amazed me how many inappropriate comments/remarks were made and have continued to be made over the course of this experience. It is also remarkable how little understanding friends and relatives have of epilepsy. Her mom suggested more rest as the panacea – as if uncontrolled seizures can be controlled by simply resting. If Susan discovered something that made a difference in her seizure activity she would be first to do it.

One comment heard often was "It could have been worse; at least you will be able to see Matthew grow up." No doubt this is true, extensive brain damage, wheelchair bound, and death could have made things worse, but Susan's response to this observation is typically "Well this is as bad as I ever want it to be." As for seeing Matthew grow up, Susan had hoped to have a more active participation in his experiences rather than what she is able to do – she has made it a goal to do as much as she can whenever she can. Having said this, participation in this manner was unexpected.

Obviously Matthew participates in life (rides a bike, swims, kicks a soccer ball, etc.). A passive observer is not the way Susan expected mothering to be. There are lost experiences with Matthew and future lost experiences to come. Each loss is difficult. When the lady who helped us in the years after the stroke would do something with Matthew it made this lost opportunity all the more painful. If Maria took Matthew to the pool or park, should Susan go along on the scooter and watch him swim or play on the swing at the park, or should she stay home and imagine the fun he was having or miss the first time he put his face in the water. Susan would go along to be present and to watch over him. This however, was never the plan. As much as possible we try to do such activities together. Matthew had his first swim lesson in the evening so I could take him into the pool and Susan could participate and enjoy this experience since it was us not an outsider.

These examples of painful choices were routinely experienced, multiple times a day, in Matthew's early years. If he fell and cried Susan could not pick him up or comfort him. As a baby, she couldn't walk with him or do any of the things that could soothe him when he was upset.

Nevertheless the goal was to be his Mom, no matter what. I normally assisted in giving him a bath, Susan selected his clothes and got down on her knees (not easy to do) to lean over the tub to wash him. What I could have done in 15 minutes might take 30 minutes. So what. If we had anything, it was time.

My assistance to facilitate her participating or doing the task, like feeding, bathing, etc., was how we operated while he was young. With the start of school there were a different set of tasks to address and we simply adapted. Susan was a room mom. Many things had to be done to arrange a party or participate in a school event. We did what had to be done so Susan could do whatever she was capable of doing.

While Susan never believed "motherhood" would be like it is, she nevertheless tries to make motherhood all that she can make it be. This gap between the expectations of what something would be like, vs. the reality of what it actually turned out to be, provided a marker for what had been lost as well as progress that had been achieved. For example, Matthew was in preschool for three years before starting kindergarten. It wasn't until the last year of preschool that Susan was able to participate in a "Mother-Child" day, by herself alone with Matthew. In fact Matthew had informed his teacher that his mom would not be able to attend this special day "because she is sick and my Dad has to go everywhere with her." He was very pleased Susan could and did attend and extremely surprised she could have done this.

Children can size situations quickly and rather accurately. Matthew knew that his mom was not like other moms, but never made anything of it, he knew nothing else. But at school he could see that there were differences between Susan and the other moms.

At some level of awareness we all know that this is the situation and it will likely never change (barring a cure for epilepsy, and reversing the damage caused by the stroke). So, rather than be negative we choose to do what we can and move on. When known obstacles are in our path, we just figure out how to avoid them and keep moving forward.

Susan's life is an example of what can be done in spite of a disability and a debilitating chronic illness. It is a testament to her deep determination and sense of independence that she sees no obstacles to the things she wants to accomplish.

Her illness is not an excuse for anything. There have been many times when it would have been easier not to do something or not to push herself. To do less or to have her epilepsy take more from her than it already has, is not Susan. She is uncompromising with regard to living her life as fully and independently as possible. Susan lives her life and refuses to have her life defined by epilepsy.

Hope is an interesting idea. I am not sure exactly what it is or how one acquires it. Hope is central to humanness. It provides a light when times are dark. It renews the spirit to continue the fight. It serves to reaffirm the importance of one's dream. Hope is at least this but in Susan's case it is the essence of who she is.

Barriers are to be overcome. Challenges are to be addressed head on and defeated. Societal (and individual's) false impressions of limited capabilities have to be confronted, dispelled, and vigorously refuted through actions and behaviors.

Unfortunately, people with a disability often confront barriers at all levels: physical, social, economic and personally. It is as if the person with a disability has to "prove" their capabilities to a level not expected of others.

Susan survived – against insurmountable odds. More than one physician has commented regarding their astonishment that Susan lived. Susan not only survived but she has thrived. She is not a disabled person but a person with a disability. She is a person with aspirations, hopes, expectations; she has a present and future perspective. The disability did not rob her of these aspirations. She would not allow that.

While Susan has physical limitations and some cognitive difficulties, she is still Susan. - an informed, interesting, and caring person. The disability did not rob her of who she is - her essence.

Make no mistake about it, life would be easier if her health were better, and the future, while perhaps unknown, would clearly be less uncertain than what we face today. The Mel Brooks movie, "High Anxiety" is an accurate characterization of our life. While the level of anxiety varies, its presence is fairly constant.

Yet Susan can smile and enjoy a good laugh. She moves forward each day, for to not do so would mean we are losing ground, missing opportunities and experiences. Take then while the taking is there.

Epilepsy is a disruption to her life; it does not define or determine it. Susan will not allow the illness to define her or become her identity. It is something she has. It is what it is. Epilepsy, in spite of its pervasive consequences on her life, does not control her life. She has it. It does not have her.

Such a description and view of herself and her world contributes to her positive and hopeful outlook on life and living. Hope is her compass, steering her life course. Neither past difficulties nor future uncertainties will throw her off course. She has a life to live, to share with others, to raise our son and to be my partner wherever this journey takes us. We are enjoying the ride!

ADDITIONAL RESOURCES

National Institute of Neurological Disorders and Stroke (NINDS)
www.NINDS.NIH.GOV
The mission of NINDS is to reduce the burden of neurological disease – a burden borne by every age group, by every segment of society, by people all over the world.

Epilepsy Foundation
www.epilepsyfoundation.org
The Epilepsy Foundation will ensure that people with seizures are able to participate in all life experiences; and will prevent, control and cure epilepsy through research, education, advocacy and services.

Citizens United for Research in Epilepsy (CURE)
www.cureepilepsy.org
CURE is a volunteer-based nonprofit organization founded by parents of children with epilepsy. It is dedicated to finding a cure for epilepsy by raising funds for research and by increasing awareness of the prevalence and devastation of this disease.
Susan Axelrod, President & Co-Founder
Contact 800-765-7118 or 312-255-1801

American Epilepsy Society
www.AESNET.org
The American Epilepsy Society promotes research and education for professionals dedicated to the prevention, treatment and cure of epilepsy. Membership in the Society is made up of clinicians and researchers investigating basic and clinical aspects of epilepsy, and other health-care professionals interested in seizure disorders.

American Stroke Association
www.strokeassociation.org
The American Stroke Association is the division of the American Heart Association that's solely focused on reducing disability and

death from stroke through research, education, fund raising and advocacy. The American Heart Association created the American Stroke Association after many years of increasing emphasis on stroke. The American Heart Association spends more money on stroke research and programs than any other organization except the federal government.

National Stroke Association

www.stroke.org

The mission of the National Stoke Association is to provide a range of educational programs and community based activities directed at prevention, treatment, and the rehabilitation of stroke-affected individuals and their families.

National Alliance for Caregiving

www.caregiving.org

The National Alliance for Caregiving is dedicated to providing support to family caregivers and the professionals who help them and to increasing public awareness of issues facing family caregivers.

National Family Caregiver Association

www.thefamilycaregiver.org

The National Family Caregivers Association (NFCA) supports, empowers, educates, and speaks up for the more than 50 million Americans who care for a chronically ill, aged, or disabled loved one.

Children of Aging Parents (CAPS)

www.caps4caregivers.org

CAPS is a non-profit, charitable organization whose mission is to assist the nation's nearly 54 million caregivers of the elderly and chronically ill with reliable information, referrals, and support, and to heighten public awareness that the health of the caregiver is essential to ensure quality care of the nation's growing elderly population.

CHANGED FOREVER

A STORY OF DETERMINATION, LOVE AND HOPE

CHANGED FOREVER tells the story determination, love and hope when faced with a life altering event.

At the age of 38, Susan Eik Filstead suffered a catastrophic stroke the morning after her son, Matthew, was born. Acute care, treatment and rehabilitation caused her to miss the first three-and-one half years of his life.

Her husband, Bill, describes the impact this event has had on her, their son and himself through a personal diary he has kept over the 16 years since this stroke. It is a deeply moving and personal portrayal of their love, devotion to each other, and Susan's determination. The importance of **HOPE** is told in a raw, frank and humorous manner. As Bill points out, "Either we either can cry or laugh at the mess we are in—we choose to laugh. Without laughter we would have been dead a while ago."

Bill's story of Susan's relentless effort to regain her life, to re-learn basic skills and tasks we all take for granted and her unwavering desire to walk and be recognized as Matthew's Mom and Bill's wife, will inspire you.

Susan lives with hope! Those who read this book will discover that "anything is possible," and will be renewed with a sense of hope to move forward and confront the challenges in their lives.

ABOUT THE AUTHOR:

Bill Filstead has advanced degrees in sociology and teaches sociology and conducts health related research. He lives in Arlington Heights, Illinois, with Susan and his son, Matthew, as well as his two older daughters who live nearby.

Made in the USA
Middletown, DE
25 October 2023

41399378R00176